Omega-3 acid ethyl esters for secondary prevention post-myocardial infarction

UK edition

CN Verboom
Solvay Pharmaceuticals, Hannover, Germany

R Marchioli
Laboratory of Clinical Epidemiology of Cardiovascular Disease,
Consorzio Mario Negri Sud, Santa Maria Imbaro, Italy

H Rupp
Molecular Cardiology Laboratory, Department of Internal Medicine and Cardiology,
Philipps University of Marburg, Marburg, Germany

B Jäger
Solvay Pharmaceuticals, Hannover, Germany

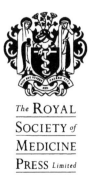

The ROYAL
SOCIETY *of*
MEDICINE
PRESS *Limited*

This monograph is published by the Royal Society of Medicine Press Ltd with financial support from the sponsor. The editors are responsible for the scientific content and for the views expressed, which are not necessarily those of the sponsor, of the Royal Society of Medicine or of the Royal Society of Medicine Press Ltd. The relevant pharmaceutical manufacturer's Data Sheets should be referred to before prescribing any of the drugs discussed in the following pages. Distribution has been in accordance with the wishes of the sponsor.

Sponsored by an educational grant from
Solvay Healthcare Ltd, Southampton, UK

British Library Cataloguing in Publication Data
A catalogue record for this book is available from the British Library

ISBN 1-85315-563-2

Text development by Hughes Associates, 3 Collins Street, Oxford, OX4 1XS

Phototypeset by Phoenix Photosetting, Chatham, Kent
Printed in Great Britain by Ebenezer Baylis, The Trinity Press, Worcester

Contents

Preface

Although great progress has been made in the prevention of cardiovascular death, the mortality of patients who survive a myocardial infarction (MI) remains high. One of the major factors contributing to this situation is sudden death. Nearly half of the cardiovascular deaths in the USA each year are attributed to this unpredictable and unexpected cause. There is thus a clear medical need for therapies targeted at reducing the incidence of sudden death in patients following an MI.

The pathological substrate of sudden death is the electrical instability of the surviving myocardium. Because of the loss of viable tissue, the surviving myocardium becomes hypertrophied and is affected by an enhanced neuro-endocrine drive. One of the consequences is an adverse remodelling of not only the extracellular matrix but also the cardiocyte itself. Any fibrosis impairs the coronary perfusion further, thereby amplifying the risk of re-infarction.

In view of the diverse pathophysiological processes involved, it may be anticipated that a comprehensive strategy for secondary prevention requires combination therapy. Current therapies partially target disorders that favour electrical instability: angiotensin-converting enzyme (ACE) inhibitors counteract adverse remodelling processes, beta-blockers reduce enhanced adrenergic influences resulting from impaired heart function, and antiplatelet agents (eg aspirin and possibly statins) reduce the occurrence of ischaemic events. It appears, however, that a therapy targeted at cardiac membrane lipids in the infarcted heart has not received adequate attention.

Membranes are an integral part of cardiocytes and conducting cells. The lipid structure of membranes is not a static property. As in the case of proteins, individual fatty acids within membranes exhibit a turnover. It has been a misconception that fatty acids in membranes can be exchanged without altering the function of embedded proteins, such as ion channels, ion pumps, ion exchangers, receptors and other signalling systems. Whereas efforts related to altering the expression of channel proteins have not yet come up with a practical approach for preventing re-infarction, studies focusing on membrane lipids have been successful. Experiments have shown that ischaemia-induced electrical instability of the heart can be reduced by incorporating long-chain omega-3 polyunsaturated fatty acids (PUFAs) into cardiac membranes.

This therapeutic approach has become of particular interest because the amount of omega-3 PUFAs required for observing an increase in electrical stability is low in humans. This is demonstrated clearly by the Gruppo Italiano per lo Studio della Sopravvivenza nell'Infarto miocardico (GISSI)-Prevenzione trial, in which Omacor (1 g/day: 90% acid ethyl esters of omega-3 PUFAs) had a substantial clinical benefit, saving lives in patients surviving an MI.

This important new treatment is described in this monograph and is examined in the context of other therapies for the secondary prevention of MI.

Heinz Rupp, PhD, Professor of Physiology, Molecular Cardiology Laboratory, Department of Internal Medicine and Cardiology, Philipps University of Marburg, Marburg, Germany

Abbreviations

Note: study acronyms are defined in Appendix 1 on p 41.

ACE	Angiotensin-converting enzyme
CHO	Chinese hamster ovary
DBSA	Delipidated bovine serum albumin
DHA	Docosahexaenoic acid
ECG	Electrocardiogram
EPA	Eicosapentaenoic acid
HDL	High-density lipoprotein
HRV	Heart rate variability
ICD	Implantable cardioverter-defibrillator
LDL	Low-density lipoprotein
MI	Myocardial infarction
NNT	Number of patients that need to be treated to prevent one death
PAI-1	Plasminogen activator inhibitor 1
PROBE	Prospective, randomized, open, with blinded endpoint evaluation
PUFA	Polyunsaturated fatty acid
VPC	Ventricular premature complex

1 Introduction

Enormous progress has been made in the management of acute myocardial infarction (MI) in the past 35 years [1]. The evolution of coronary care units and of public and physician education to encourage rapid response, the development of catheter-based revascularization techniques, and a greater emphasis on cardiac rehabilitation have all contributed to improvements in the prognosis of MI patients.

By common agreement, however, one of the most significant factors contributing to this progress has been the development, through controlled clinical trials, of an extensive and well-proven repertoire of medical therapies. The use of intravenous thrombolytics, aspirin, beta-blockers and angiotensin-converting enzyme (ACE) inhibitors has had a transforming influence on the immediate- and longer-term prospects for MI patients. The success of these measures has been described in various surveys of mortality trends, with progressive reductions in both short-term (28-day) and intermediate-term (two–three-year) mortality rates among MI patients [2–6].

Patients who have survived an acute MI are nevertheless a high-risk group, with a life expectancy sometimes half that of their peers who have not experienced a similar event [6] and with a greatly increased risk for subsequent major cardiovascular events and death [7, 8]. To the extent that patients who have suffered a first MI are at greater risk for subsequent infarction, diminished life expectancy may reflect imperfect implementation of secondary prevention strategies [9, 10]. It is likely, however, that sudden cardiac death is a major contributor to this situation [11]. Sudden death has proved resistant to therapeutic innovation to a greater degree than atherothrombotic coronary disease. Incidence rates of sudden death post-MI have declined during the era of thrombolytic therapy, but they remain as high as 5% in the two and a half years after an index MI [12] and are certainly substantially higher than in the general population (Figure 1). Nearly half the cardiovascular deaths in the USA each year are attributed to this cause [13, 14]. The current expert perspective on sudden death related to coronary disease is that it is 'the single most important cause of death in the adult population of the industrialized world' [12].

Impressive results in the prevention of sudden death have been achieved with implantable cardioverter-defibrillators (ICDs) [15–18] (Figure 1). Mortality data confirm a benefit from these devices in closely defined groups of high-risk patients. In several instances, these data were obtained in trials versus drug therapies, which highlights the paucity of medical options in this area of medicine [19–21]. However, no similar trial of ICDs has been undertaken in unselected MI patients, and even if such a study were undertaken (which is not likely) and a benefit was proven (also not certain), then the cost of these devices would almost certainly preclude their general use in the post-MI population. (See, for example, Coletta et al. [18] for cost estimates for

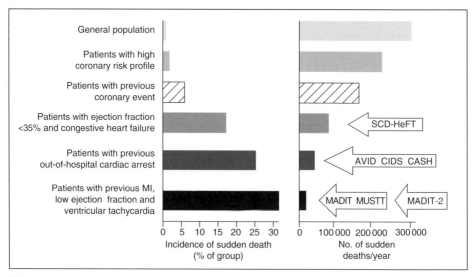

Figure 1 Incidence of sudden death and numbers of sudden death events in different patient populations. Acronyms in arrows indicate trials in high-risk patients in which ICDs have been shown to have survival benefits.

Reproduced with permission from Myerburg et al. [15], with additions.

treating only that proportion of patients who meet the eligibility criteria for MADIT-2.)*

The need for an effective, easy-to-use, broadly applicable, affordable medical therapy to prevent sudden death is thus clear. A candidate therapy has emerged recently in the form of concentrated and highly purified omega-3 polyunsaturated fatty acids (omega-3 [or n-3] PUFAs). In the GISSI-Prevenzione study, use of highly purified omega-3 PUFAs in the form of Omacor 1 g/day was associated with a 45% reduction in the risk of sudden death [22, 23]. This is an effect size that exceeds that of any other medical therapy studied for the impact on sudden death (Table 1) and, importantly [12], was recorded in a trial in which total mortality was reduced significantly [22–24].

The results of the GISSI-Prevenzione study identified Omacor as an important addition to the armamentarium for secondary prevention post-MI. Omacor addresses a major unmet need. It is administered easily and tolerated well and it is appropriate for the general population of post-MI patients. On the basis of the GISSI-Prevenzione trial results, Omacor has been registered as 'adjuvant treatment in secondary prevention after myocardial infarction, in addition to other standard therapy' in several countries [25]. This monograph reviews the clinical evidence for the use of Omacor to save lives in post-MI patients and considers the possible mechanisms of action that underpin these benefits.

*Another recent perspective on the potential of public access defibrillation and its realizability has been published by Weaver WD and Peberdy MA. N Engl J Med 2002; **347**: 1223–4.

Drug category	No. of patients	Relative risk of death (95% CI)	Relative risk of SCD (95% CI)
Omacor	11 324	0.80 (0.67–0.94)*	0.55 (0.40–0.76)
ACE inhibitors post-MI	15 104	0.83 (0.71–0.97)	0.80 (0.70–0.92)
Aldosterone receptor blockers	1663	0.70 (0.60–0.82)	0.71 (0.54–0.95)
Sodium channel blockers post-MI**	>23 000		>1.0
Flecainide/encainide***	1455		3.6 (1.7–8.5)
Beta-blockers post-MI**, ****	24 298		0.77 (0.70–0.84)
Amiodarone**	6500		0.71 (0.59–0.85)
d-Sotalol	3121		1.77 (1.15–2.74)
Calcium channel blockers**	20 342		1.04 (0.95–1.14)

Table 1 The effect of various drug categories on sudden cardiac death (SCD). The reduction in SCD achieved with Omacor in the GISSI-Prevenzione study is the largest such benefit seen with a medical intervention in post-MI patients without overt heart failure. (Results of studies involving patients with heart failure are not summarized in this table.)

Data from Priori *et al.* [12] and GISSI-Prevenzione Investigators [22].
*Death from all causes tested as one or more combined parameters accounting for the study's primary endpoint.
**Includes data from meta-analyses.
***Data on SCD from CAST.
****Not including specific studies of, for example, carvedilol and metoprolol in patients with heart failure.

2 Introduction to Omacor

Omacor is a pharmaceutical preparation of highly purified and concentrated omega-3 PUFAs containing 90% omega-3 PUFAs per 1 g. Almost all (84%) the PUFA content of Omacor is docosahexaenoic acid (DHA) and eicosapentaenoic acid (EPA) (Figure 2). Omacor administered at a dose of 1 g/day has been approved for secondary prevention post-MI on the basis of the results of the GISSI-Prevenzione trial, a large, multicentre study conducted in more than 11 000 patients. The GISSI-Prevenzione study is examined in detail in the next chapter.

2.1 FATTY ACID NOTATION

The active ingredients of Omacor are referred to as omega-3 PUFAs because of their distinctive physical and structural chemistry. Fatty acids may be classified according to the length of the aliphatic carbon chain and the number (if any) and location of double bonds within that chain, counting from the omega (or n) terminal [26]. Thus, for example, a fatty acid with an 18-carbon chain and no double bonds would be classified as *c18*. A similar compound with two double bonds would be classified as *c18:2 (n-x)*. The number after the colon signifies the number of double bonds, and the term in parentheses indicates at which carbon atom from the omega-terminal the first double bond is encountered. If the molecule had three double bonds, the first occurring at the omega-3 position, then the notation would be *c18:3 (n-3)*.

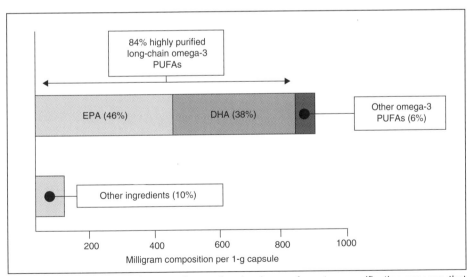

Figure 2 Composition of Omacor. Preparation involves a four-stage purification process that eliminates a range of impurities and minimizes the content of saturated fats.

Types of fatty acids recognized in this notation include *saturates*, such as stearic acid and palmitic acid, *monounsaturates*, exemplified by oleic acid, and two major classes of *polyunsaturated fatty acids* (Figure 3).

Omega-6 polyunsaturated fatty acids (omega-6 PUFAs) have multiple double bonds, the first of which occurs at the omega-6 position. The most abundant of the omega-6 PUFAs found in the diet is linoleic acid (*c18:2 [n-6]*). Arguably the most important product of linoleic acid metabolism is arachidonic acid (*c20:4 [n-6]*) (Figure 3), the substrate for the classic prostaglandin cascade.

In *omega-3 polyunsaturated fatty acids* (omega-3 PUFAs), the first of the multiple double bonds occurs at the omega-3 position (Figure 3). The short-chain omega-3 PUFA alpha-linolenic acid (*c18:2 [n-3]*) can be derived from dietary sources, such as dried butternut, raw soya beans and leeks. The longer-chain omega-3 PUFAs, DHA and EPA, may be synthesized from alpha-linolenic acid in mammalian cells [27]. There appears to be only limited capacity for synthesis of EPA and DHA from alpha-linolenic acid [28], however, so EPA and DHA must be obtained from exogenous sources if they are to be available in sufficient quantities for physiological needs. Moreover, because the turnover of membrane fatty acids is accelerated by a high sympathetic activity, the supply of essential fatty acids such as omega-3 PUFAs has to occur regularly and in adequate amounts to ensure their continuous presence in membranes [29, 30]. Omacor provides a simple solution to the need for a reliable source of long-chain omega-3 PUFAs.

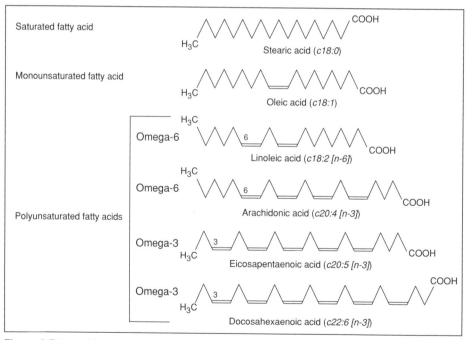

Figure 3 Fatty acid nomenclature. These compounds are classified according to their degree of saturation/unsaturation and the position of any double bonds.

3 The GISSI-Prevenzione Trial

3.1 GISSI-PREVENZIONE: OVERVIEW

GISSI-Prevenzione was an investigator-led multicentre study undertaken to examine the impact of Omacor on outcomes post-MI in the context of contemporary preventive practice. The study was therefore designed to be as inclusive as possible. No age limits were specified, and exclusion criteria were kept to a minimum. Patients with a recent MI (three months or less) were eligible to participate in the study provided they had no condition associated with poor short-term prognosis (including, but not limited to, severe congestive heart failure and cancer), no known contraindications to the study medications, and no known congenital coagulation defect [22].

Drugs for secondary prevention (eg antiplatelet drugs, beta-blockers, ACE inhibitors) were recommended according to prevailing standard practice. In addition, patients were encouraged to adhere to recommended preventive measures, including a Mediterranean-style diet with a high content of fruit, fish and fibre, and a relatively low content of saturated fats.

A total of 11 324 patients were recruited and randomized at 172 centres, making GISSI-Prevenzione one of the larger studies in secondary prevention. Information on end-of-study vital status was recorded for 99.9% of participants, yielding more than 38 000 patient-years of data during an average three and a half years of follow-up.

Treatment assignment is summarized in Figure 4. Study medications comprised Omacor, administered at a dose of 1 g/day and comprising 84% EPA and DHA, and vitamin E, administered as alpha-tocopherol 300 mg/day. Treatments were administered open-

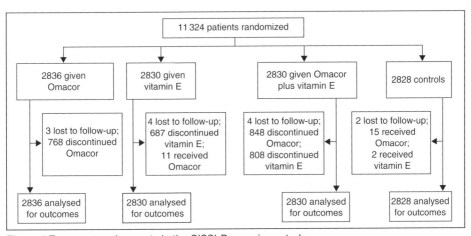

Figure 4 Treatment assignments in the GISSI-Prevenzione study.

label, with ascertainment of prospectively defined endpoints by a blinded endpoint validation committee. This prospective, randomized, open, with blinded endpoint evaluation (PROBE) format has been used in other major cardiovascular trials, such as the HOT study [31].

Baseline characteristics of participating patients are shown in Table 2 [22]. Features worthy of comment include the relatively low proportions of elderly patients (16% >70 years old) and patients with a low ejection fraction or evidence of active ischaemia during stress testing. (The small proportion of patients with a low ejection fraction [~14% with an ejection fraction ≤40%] was a consequence of the exclusion of patients with overt heart failure.) Average baseline lipoprotein levels were higher than would be considered desirable for post-MI patients [32], but the use of recommended preventive therapies at baseline was generally high, particularly in the case of antiplatelet agents. Lipid-lowering drugs were not recommended therapies when the GISSI-Prevenzione study was initiated, but the publication of several pivotal trials of statins during the mid-1990s led to the assimilation of these agents into standard practice at participating centres during subsequent years. This evolution in secondary preventive strategy was reflected in the usage rates of statins in the Omacor cohort, which increased from less than 5% at the start of GISSI-Prevenzione to nearly 50% at completion of follow-up. This increasing use of statins during the trial is unlikely to have influenced the results of the study, however, as usage increased in a similar manner in all treatment groups.

Adherence to the advised diet, as represented by patient-reported consumption of sentinel foodstuffs, was high throughout the study and tended to improve with duration of follow-up (Table 3) [22].

3.2 STUDY ENDPOINTS

The GISSI-Prevenzione study had two prespecified primary efficacy endpoints:

- cumulative rate of all-cause mortality, nonfatal MI and nonfatal stroke;
- cumulative rate of cardiovascular mortality, nonfatal MI and nonfatal stroke.

Fatal endpoint definitions were based on a nested ('Russian doll') classification (Figure 5).

A nonfatal MI was diagnosed when a patient exhibited any two of:

- pathognomonic chest pain;
- ST changes of 1 mm or more in any limb lead, or of more than 2 mm in any precordial lead, or both;
- a doubling or greater increase in diagnostic enzymes.

A nonfatal stroke was diagnosed if a patient exhibited unequivocal signs or symptoms of persisting neurological deficit with a sudden onset and duration of at least 24 hours.

Secondary efficacy analyses included inspection of all components of the primary endpoints and the principal causes of death.

3.3 STATISTICAL CONSIDERATIONS AND METHODS

Statistical calculations were based on the assumptions that the cumulative

Characteristic	Omacor (n = 2836)	Vitamin E (n = 2830)	Omacor plus vitamin E (n = 2830)	Controls (n = 2828)
Male	2403 (84.7%)	2398 (84.7%)	2451 (86.6%)	2407 (85.1%)
Female	433 (15.3%)	432 (15.3%)	379 (13.3%)	421 (14.9%)
Mean (SD) characteristics				
Age (years)	59.4 (10.7)	59.5 (10.5)	59.1 (10.5)	59.4 (10.5)
Days since diagnosis of acute MI	25.4 (21.0)	25.0 (20.7)	24.7 (20.7)	25.2 (21.1)
Body mass index (kg/m²)	26.5 (3.9)	26.5 (3.6)	26.6 (3.6)	26.4 (3.5)
Ejection fraction (%)	52.6 (10.6)	52.9 (10.5)	52.4 (10.5)	52.5 (10.8)
Total blood cholesterol (mg/dl)	210.2 (42.1)	211.1 (42.4)	210.6 (41.5)	211.6 (42.3)
LDL cholesterol (mg/dl)	137.3 (39.1)	138.0 (38.1)	138.2 (38.1)	138.5 (37.6)
HDL cholesterol (mg/dl)	41.5 (11.3)	41.3 (11.2)	41.6 (11.5)	41.7 (12.0)
Triglycerides (mg/dl)	162.6 (81.7)	163.3 (85.3)	160.3 (80.3)	161.9 (94.5)
Secondary diagnoses				
Arterial hypertension	1019 (36.0%)	1007 (35.6%)	1033 (36.5%)	967 (34.2%)
Diabetes mellitus	405 (14.2%)	426 (15.0%)	426 (15.0%)	426 (15.0%)
Nonsmokers	632 (22.4%)	636 (22.6%)	618 (22.0%)	613 (21.9%)
Ex-smokers	996 (35.4%)	1016 (36.1%)	972 (34.5%)	953 (34.0%)
Smokers	1189 (42.2%)	1161 (41.3%)	1223 (43.5%)	1234 (44.0%)
Body mass index ≥30 kg/m²	419 (14.7%)	403 (14.2%)	432 (15.2%)	390 (13.8%)
Ejection fraction (%)				
≤30	56 (2.3%)	69 (2.9%)	59 (2.5%)	65 (2.7%)
31–40	283 (11.7%)	245 (10.2%)	279 (11.6%)	264 (11.0%)
>40	2089 (86.0%)	2092 (87.0%)	2059 (85.9%)	2079 (86.3%)
Premature ventricular beats >10/h	259 (13.1%)	252 (12.6%)	278 (14.1%)	279 (14.1%)
Previous sustained ventricular tachycardia	17 (0.9%)	25 (1.3%)	18 (0.9%)	13 (0.7%)
Ventricular arrhythmias	373 (18.8%)	376 (18.7%)	400 (20.2%)	385 (19.4%)
Positive exercise-stress test	550 (29.8%)	511 (27.8%)	542 (29.0%)	534 (29.0%)
Pharmacological therapy				
Antiplatelet drugs				
Baseline	2601 (92.2%)	2565 (91.2%)	2582 (91.8%)	2562 (91.5%)
6 months	2308 (88.2%)	2262 (87.4%)	2261 (87.5%)	2267 (88.3%)
42 months	1707 (83.4%)	1649 (82.5%)	1685 (83.2%)	1627 (82.1%)
ACE inhibitors				
Baseline	1298 (46.0%)	1287 (45.7%)	1352 (48.1%)	1343 (48.0%)
6 months	1033 (39.5%)	1074 (41.5%)	1045 (40.4%)	1083 (42.2%)
42 months	788 (38.5%)	774 (38.7%)	826 (40.8%)	754 (38.0%)
Beta-blockers				
Baseline	1237 (43.9%)	1261 (44.8%)	1250 (44.4%)	1238 (44.2%)
6 months	1092 (41.7%)	1085 (41.9%)	1052 (40.7%)	1043 (40.6%)
42 months	807 (39.4%)	792 (39.5%)	764 (37.7%)	738 (37.2%)
Cholesterol-lowering drugs				
Baseline	124 (4.4%)	130 (4.6%)	135 (4.8%)	145 (5.1%)
6 months	782 (28.6%)	780 (28.8%)	757 (27.9%)	786 (29.1%)
42 months	1003 (46.0%)	962 (44.8%)	1013 (46.7%)	941 (44.4%)

Table 2 Baseline characteristics of patients in the GISSI-Prevenzione study.

Data from GISSI-Prevenzione Investigators [22]. HDL, high-density lipoprotein; LDL, low-density lipoprotein.

Dietary item	Omacor (n = 2836)	Vitamin E (n = 2830)	Omacor plus vitamin E (n = 2830)	Controls (n = 2828)
Fruit (≥1 per day)				
Baseline	2243 (79.9%)	2269 (80.8%)	2239 (79.8%)	2259 (80.9%)
6 months	2185 (86.7%)	2169 (87.4%)	2181 (88.4%)	2145 (86.7%)
42 months	1670 (87.9%)	1625 (88.0%)	1635 (87.5%)	1590 (88.5%)
Fresh vegetables (≥1 per day)				
Baseline	1121 (39.8%)	1088 (38.7%)	1145 (40.8%)	1107 (39.6%)
6 months	1341 (53.0%)	1299 (52.1%)	1333 (53.8%)	1331 (53.4%)
42 months	1055 (55.1%)	1010 (54.4%)	1026 (54.6%)	988 (54.4%)
Olive oil (regularly)				
Baseline	2092 (74.3%)	2085 (74.3%)	2016 (71.8%)	2066 (73.9%)
6 months	1998 (79.1%)	1993 (80.2%)	1955 (79.0%)	1990 (80.0%)
42 months	1566 (82.2%)	1542 (83.4%)	1542 (82.5%)	1486 (82.0%)
Fish (≥1 per week)				
Baseline	2050 (72.9%)	2053 (73.1%)	2057 (73.3%)	2053 (73.4%)
6 months	2170 (85.9%)	2184 (87.7%)	2137 (86.2%)	2125 (85.5%)
42 months	1676 (87.7%)	1622 (87.5%)	1651 (88.1%)	1578 (87.2%)

Table 3 Dietary habits of patients in the GISSI-Prevenzione study. Adherence to a Mediterranean-type diet was high throughout follow-up.

Data from GISSI-Prevenzione Investigators [22].

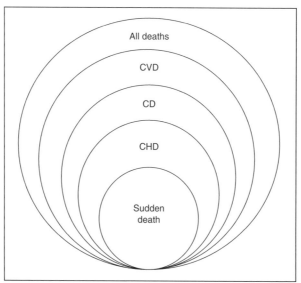

Figure 5 Interrelationships of fatal endpoints in the GISSI-Prevenzione study. All endpoints were confirmed by a blinded endpoint validation committee.

Data from GISSI-Prevenzione Investigators [22]. CVD, cardiovascular death (any cardiovascular cause); CD, cardiac death (any cardiac cause); CHD, coronary death (any coronary cause).

event rate for the primary endpoint of all-cause mortality plus nonfatal MI and nonfatal stroke would be 20% in the control group during the anticipated follow-up interval of 42 months and that the recruitment of approximately 3000 patients per group would endow the study with: (1) sufficient statistical power to discern a 20% relative risk reduction for that primary endpoint in any of the three treatment groups compared with the control group; and (2) sufficient statistical power to discern a 20% relative risk reduction for that primary endpoint with combined therapy versus either monotherapy.

Statistical comparisons emphasized four-way analysis, in which any treatment assignment could be compared with any other. Outcomes were analysed according to the principles of intention-to-treat.

3.4 PRIMARY RESULTS

3.4.1 Effects of Omacor

Omacor reduced significantly the risk of experiencing a primary endpoint event in the GISSI-Prevenzione study. Compared with controls, the risk reduction for the endpoint of all-cause mortality plus nonfatal MI and nonfatal stroke was 16% ($p = 0.02$); the risk reduction for cardiovascular death plus nonfatal MI and nonfatal stroke was 20% ($p = 0.009$) [22]. The survival benefit seen with omega-3 PUFAs during the GISSI-Prevenzione study emerged within a few months and was then sustained throughout follow-up (Figure 6).

Analysis of cause-specific mortality revealed that the prevention of primary endpoint events by Omacor was due to a reduction in all-cause mortality

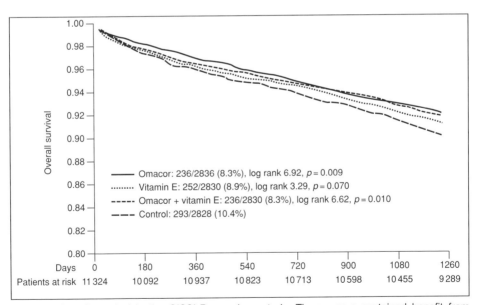

Figure 6 Overall survival in the GISSI-Prevenzione study. There was a sustained benefit from Omacor, with evidence of a treatment effect within the first few months of the study.

Reproduced with permission from GISSI-Prevenzione Investigators [22].

(20% risk reduction) and in several categories of cardiovascular death, notably sudden death (45% risk reduction) [22]. There was no significant impact on patients' risk of experiencing a nonfatal MI or nonfatal stroke (Table 4).

The findings of the secondary endpoint analysis and the observation that the risk of a primary endpoint event was reduced within a few months of starting Omacor therapy stimulated a further analysis of factors contributing to this result [23]. A re-evaluation of all fatal outcomes was therefore undertaken, blinded to treatment assignment but with the aid of event data that became available after the completion of the primary analysis. Early trends in the various forms of cardiovascular mortality were examined in detail by right-censoring survival data at monthly intervals beginning at the first month after randomization. This analysis confirmed an early treatment benefit on total survival that was significantly different from that in the control group after three months (41% risk reduction; $p = 0.037$) and thereafter remained statistically significant and clinically meaningful for the remainder of the study (Figure 7a) [23]. The re-evaluation procedure confirmed 265 cases of sudden death during the study. A similar censored analysis of these events revealed an early effect of Omacor in reducing the risk of sudden death, with a large (53%) and statistically significant ($p = 0.048$) benefit

Outcomes	Omacor (n = 2836)	Controls (n = 2828)	Omacor relative risk (95% CI)
Main endpoints			
Death, nonfatal MI and nonfatal stroke	356 (12.3%)	414 (14.6%)	0.85 (0.74–0.98)
CVD death, nonfatal MI and nonfatal stroke	262 (9.2%)	322 (11.4%)	0.80 (0.68–0.95)
Secondary analyses			
All fatal events	236 (8.3%)	293 (10.4%)	0.80 (0.67–0.94)
CVD death	136 (4.8%)	193 (6.8%)	0.70 (0.56–0.87)
Cardiac death	108 (3.8%)	165 (5.8%)	0.65 (0.51–0.82)
Coronary death	100 (3.5%)	151 (5.3%)	0.65 (0.51–0.84)
Sudden death	55 (1.9%)	99 (3.5%)	0.55 (0.40–0.76)
Other death	100 (3.5%)	100 (3.5%)	0.99 (0.75–1.30)
Nonfatal CVD events	140 (4.9%)	144 (5.1%)	0.96 (0.76–1.21)
Subsidiary analyses			
CHD death and nonfatal MI	196 (6.9%)	259 (9.2%)	0.75 (0.62–0.90)
Fatal and nonfatal stroke	54 (1.9%)	41 (1.5%)	1.30 (0.87–1.96)

Table 4 Summary of primary and secondary endpoint results in the GISSI-Prevenzione study. Data are derived from four-way analysis. Patients with two or more events of different types appear more than once in columns but only once in rows.

Data from GISSI-Prevenzione Investigators [22]. CHD, coronary death; CVD, cardiovascular death.

apparent after four months (Figure 7b) [23]. The reduction in sudden death at three months, although not statistically significant ($p = 0.058$), accounted for more than half of the reduction in total mortality at that time. By the end of follow-up, the reduction in sudden death was highly statistically significant ($p = 0.0006$) and accounted for 59% of the total survival benefit of Omacor versus controls.

Significant ($p \leq 0.05$) reductions in the risk of cardiovascular, cardiac and coronary deaths were achieved after six to nine months of treatment with Omacor. The reduction in risk of both combined primary endpoint events (all-cause mortality plus nonfatal MI and nonfatal stroke, and cardiovascular mortality plus nonfatal MI and nonfatal stroke) became statistically significant at nine months. The time course of treatment effects is summarized in Table 5.

These data were interpreted by the investigators as confirmation that much of the benefit of Omacor seen in the GISSI-Prevenzione study was attributable to an early and then sustained effect to prevent sudden death.

Combined therapy with Omacor plus vitamin E had effects similar to those of Omacor alone. There was no indication of any clinical synergism between the two treatments.

3.4.2 Lipoprotein and biochemistry effects

Comparison of cholesterol and triglyceride data at baseline and after six months of treatment revealed no substantial effects of Omacor on these parameters at the dose administered in the trial. Control-adjusted levels of cholesterol lipoproteins did not change by more than 2.5%, and triglyceride levels were reduced by less than 5% relative to the control group. Blood glucose levels and fibrinogen concentrations were not altered substantively during therapy.

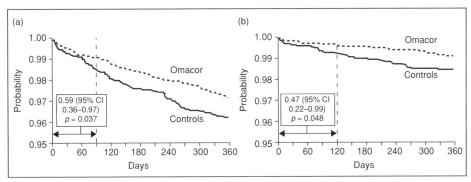

Figure 7 Effect of Omacor on risk of (a) all-cause mortality and (b) sudden death. There was evidence for a significant reduction in total mortality with highly purified omega-3 PUFAs in the GISSI-Prevenzione study after three months of treatment, and evidence of a significant reduction in sudden death after four months. Most of the early reduction in total mortality was attributable to reduction in sudden death.

Reproduced with permission from Marchioli *et al.* [23].

Outcome	Time (months)					
	3	4	6	9	12	42
Primary endpoints				✓	✓	✓
Secondary endpoints						
All-cause mortality	✓	✓	✓	✓	✓	✓
Sudden death		✓	✓	✓	✓	✓
Coronary death				✓		✓
Cardiac death			✓	✓	✓	✓
Cardiovascular death				✓	✓	✓

Table 5 Time course of mortality benefits of Omacor in the GISSI-Prevenzione study.

Data from Marchioli et al. [23].
✓ = statistically significant effect of Omacor ($p \leq 0.05$).

3.4.3 Tolerability and safety

Omacor was tolerated well during the study. Gastrointestinal disturbances and nausea were the main adverse events reported during the study, and the rate of discontinuation for treatment-related adverse events was very low (Table 6) [22]. Numbers of deaths due to noncardiovascular causes were similar in both the Omacor group and the control group. This category of events therefore made no contribution to the superiority of Omacor over controls for the primary endpoints of the GISSI-Prevenzione study. These data provided further reassurance, however, that there were no substantive noncardiovascular safety concerns for the long-term use of Omacor.

3.4.4 Effects of vitamin E

Vitamin E had no significant effect on either of the primary endpoints of the study, and, unlike Omacor, had no significant impact on all-cause mortality. Significant effects were observed on several of the secondary endpoints, but in the absence of any effect on the primary outcomes the validity and relevance of these effects are uncertain.

The rationale for anticipating a cardioprotective benefit from vitamin E in secondary prevention is that its antioxidant qualities will inhibit atherogenesis, primarily by preventing oxidative modification of low-density lipoprotein (LDL) [33]. Experience with vitamin E in the prevention of cardiovascular diseases is contradictory, however, with indications of benefit in observational studies but only limited corroboration of this in controlled trials [34]. The data from the GISSI-

Principal adverse events	
Gastrointestinal disturbances	4.9
Nausea	1.4
Discontinuation due to adverse events	3.8*
Cumulative discontinuation from therapy after 3.5 years	28.5**

Table 6 Incidence (%) of reported adverse events and rate of discontinuation related to adverse events in the GISSI-Prevenzione study.

Data from GISSI-Prevenzione Investigators [22].
*2.1% with vitamin E.
**26.2% with vitamin E.

Prevenzione study join a now substantial volume of data from other large controlled clinical trials (eg HOPE [35], HPS [36], ATBC [37]), which indicate that vitamin E offers no discernible benefit in the generality of patients with established coronary disease (including MI survivors). In HPS, for example, supplementation with vitamin E (600 mg/day for a planned five years) had no effect on total or cause-specific mortality or nonfatal cardiovascular events [36]. Those trials that have reported a benefit from vitamin E have tended to be small and have either involved specific populations (eg patients undergoing haemodialysis in the SPACE study [38]) or have identified effects on non-fatal outcomes (eg CHAOS [39]).

Available data from large clinical trials therefore do not currently support the widespread use of vitamin E in secondary prevention, but the results of trials such as GISSI-Prevenzione may reasonably be regarded as identifying hypotheses for further study. One aspect of vitamin E therapy that merits closer scrutiny is the possibility that synthetic vitamin E may differ from the natural form in ways and to an extent that compromise the potential benefit of this substance. Another possibility for consideration is that a high degree of oxidative stress (ie demand for vitamin E) rather than a high degree of supply may be a better marker of patients likely to benefit from this therapy [33, 40].

4 Perspective on Omacor

GISSI-Prevenzione is the largest clinical trial to date of the effects of highly purified omega-3 PUFAs on outcomes in post-MI patients. The benefit demonstrated with these agents in the GISSI-Prevenzione study is not, however, an isolated finding. The findings of the DART study [41], in particular, provide strong corroboration of the outcomes data from GISSI-Prevenzione.

DART was a clinical trial of factorial design conducted in 2033 nondiabetic men aged under 70 years who had recently recovered from an MI. After two years of follow-up, a significant survival benefit was recorded in men who had been instructed to augment their intake of omega-3 PUFAs (29% risk reduction; $p < 0.05$). No benefit was noted with any of the other interventions examined. The survival benefit in DART was not accompanied by any effect on risk of nonfatal events, an outcome exactly in conformity with the results of the GISSI-Prevenzione study.

Similarities between the trials are strengthened by the fact that the DART investigators attributed the net survival benefit seen in that study to an early effect of omega-3 PUFAs on reducing case-fatality rates, probably as a result of an arrhythmia-preventing action. Moreover, they subscribed to the view that omega-3 PUFAs were the active principle responsible for this effect [42].

The magnitude of the treatment effect seen in DART was broadly congruent with the results of GISSI-Prevenzione, although in a recent commentary the lead investigator of DART suggested that the difference in risk reduction for all-cause mortality (29% in DART, 20% in GISSI-Prevenzione) was sufficiently large to be indicative of a dietary influence on outcomes [42]. On first encounter, this is an interesting hypothesis: DART was conducted in the UK and many of the participants had an unsatisfactory baseline dietary profile, involving high intake of saturated and hydrogenated fats, refined sugars, etc. By contrast, patients in GISSI-Prevenzione were broadly adherent to the Mediterranean style of diet now widely recommended as an element of both primary and secondary prevention [22, 32, 42]; Omacor was used in addition to both dietary and other pharmacological measures.

There are, however, reasons to doubt this possibility. Data from the GISSI-Prevenzione study indicate that the survival benefit of Omacor in that study was greater in patients who were most closely compliant with the Mediterranean diet [43]. The pragmatic conclusion from this analysis of the GISSI-Prevenzione database is that dietary modification is a valuable discipline post-MI but that Omacor confers additional benefit, even in conditions of optimal dietary control, and represents an essential element in any comprehensive preventive strategy, irrespective of dietary habits.

Moreover, it should be recalled that there was much more widespread use of preventive medications in GISSI-Prevenzione than in DART. Such variances could contribute towards the difference in effect size for reduction in all-cause mortality between the two studies.

The scale of the treatment benefit offered by any therapy is a function of event rate in the population under consideration. Participants in the GISSI-Prevenzione study were, by the standards of post-MI patients, at relatively low risk: the annualized mortality rate in the control group was 2.8% [23]. The absolute risk reduction achieved with Omacor was 2.1% over three and a half years, yielding a number of patients that need to be treated to prevent or avoid one death (NNT) of approximately 177/year, or about six deaths prevented per 1000 patient-years of treatment. This figure would be regarded widely as a reasonable investment of effort to prevent one death. In a population with an annual mortality rate of approximately 5%, the NNT would be halved (assuming constant relative risk reduction).

Recent reports from observational studies are also supportive of a cardioprotective quality of omega-3 PUFAs. Pertinently, two of these studies – a prospective, nested case-control study undertaken as part of the US Physicians' Health Study [44] and

a case-control study of all episodes of primary cardiac arrest at two sites in the USA over a six-year period [45] – documented a marked inverse correlation between blood levels of omega-3 PUFAs [44, 45] or omega-3 PUFA intake [45] and the incidence of sudden death (Table 7). These findings are all the more noteworthy because the participants in these studies had no history of ischaemic coronary disease. Sudden death is the first clinical expression of coronary artery disease in many cases [43]. Thus, these data not only support the central GISSI-Prevenzione finding of a survival benefit due to reduced risk of sudden death, but also hint at a possible role for omega-3 PUFAs in primary prevention. Such a possibility has been acknowledged by other commentators and is currently being evaluated in a large clinical trial in primary care [46].

Strong relations between omega-3 PUFA intake and cardiovascular well-being have also been reported recently from the US Nurses' Health Study [47]. These data are notable both for relating to the risk of cardiovascular disease in women – still a relatively underinvestigated subject – and for the size and duration of the

Variable	Quartile of omega-3 PUFAs				p value for trend
	1 (lowest blood level)	2	3	4 (highest blood level)	
Relative risk of sudden death	1.0	0.55	0.28	0.19	0.007
95% CI		0.18–1.70	0.09–0.87	0.05–0.71	

Table 7 Relation between omega-3 PUFA intake and incidence of sudden death. Investigation of the relation between baseline blood levels of omega-3 PUFAs and the risk of sudden death in men with no history of coronary disease revealed a significant correlation between higher blood levels of omega-3 PUFAs and lower risk of sudden death. Data shown are from a multivariate analysis adjusting for factors including body mass index, diabetes status, family history and baseline cholesterol.

Data from Albert *et al.* [44].

survey: the most recent report draws on more than 1.3 million woman-years of follow-up over 16 years. Exact parallels cannot be drawn with the GISSI-Prevenzione study because the classification system adopted in the Nurses' Health Study precluded the identification of sudden death. Death from coronary heart disease was determined, however, and was shown to be related inversely to omega-3 PUFA intake. The age-adjusted relative risk of a fatal coronary heart disease event in the quintile with the highest omega-3 PUFA intake was 58% lower than in patients in the lowest quintile of the omega-3 PUFA intake distribution. This finding remained both large (~40%) and statistically significant ($p < 0.001$ for trend) after adjustment for multiple potential confounding factors. There was also a correlation between higher omega-3 PUFA intake and reduced risk for nonfatal coronary heart disease, although the effect size (30–40%) was consistently smaller than for fatal coronary heart disease.

Separately, Sellmayer *et al.* [48] reported a 48% reduction in ventricular premature complexes (VPCs) after 16 weeks of dietary omega-3 PUFA supplementation in patients with a history of VPCs ($p = 0.052$ versus placebo); VPCs were reduced by 70% or more in 44% of treated patients ($p < 0.01$ versus placebo).

4.1 OMACOR IN THE CONTEXT OF CURRENT SECONDARY PREVENTIVE STRATEGIES

Secondary prevention post-MI has undergone a remarkable evolution in the past two decades, due in large part to extensive clinical trials of various medical interventions. The current recommended repertoire of drug therapies for secondary prevention includes the following agents, in approximate chronological order of their evaluation in clinical trials [32, 49, 50]:

- antiplatelet agents, pre-eminently aspirin
- beta-blockers
- ACE inhibitors
- lipid-lowering drugs.

The impact of fibrinolytic therapies in MI is beyond dispute [51]. These drugs form part of the acute-phase medical response to MI, however, and will not be discussed further.

4.1.1 Antiplatelet agents

Aspirin is now such a central element in secondary prevention that it is easy to overlook the fact that the first reports of its use in this indication were statistically inconclusive and that only the sound instincts of the original investigators led to further clinical trials [52, 53]. The results of those subsequent trials established that aspirin has a profound impact on prognosis post-MI when administered at doses of 75–325 mg/day [54].

The most recent meta-analysis of the effects of antiplatelet therapy (almost exclusively aspirin) in controlled trials in secondary prevention has accumulated data from some 20 000 post-MI patients [55]. Therapy for a mean interval of 27 months was associated with a 25% reduction in risk of a vascular event, equivalent to preventing 36 such events per 1000 patients treated ($p < 0.0001$); for the endpoint of all-cause mortality, antiplatelet medication prevented 12 events per 1000 patients ($p = 0.02$).

Analysis of recent trials comparing aspirin with newer antiplatelet agents, such as clopidogrel and ticlopidine, has revealed that the latter agents may offer modest additional benefits over aspirin and are realistic alternative therapies for patients who are intolerant of aspirin. Data from direct comparative studies indicate no substantive benefit of aspirin plus dipyridamole over aspirin alone.

4.1.2 Anticoagulants

Anticoagulation as part of the secondary prevention regimen improves prognosis post-MI, but the overall scale of this benefit is not greater than that seen with aspirin [56]. For most patients, therefore, aspirin represents an easier and cheaper treatment. Anticoagulants may be considered when patients are intolerant of aspirin but, as noted above, clopidogrel may represent a more suitable alternative in many cases. Increasingly, therefore, the use of anticoagulants is restricted to patients with a propensity to thromboembolic complications. Examples include individuals with large anterior MI, left ventricular aneurysm or persistent atrial fibrillation [32, 57].

4.1.3 Beta-blockers

Evidence from clinical trials and meta-analyses indicates clearly that long-term treatment with beta-blockers is beneficial in unselected post-MI patients: the risk of all-cause mortality is reduced by 23%, an effect that equates to preventing 12 deaths per 1000 patients treated for one year [58]. This conclusion is robust, being based on data from approximately 25 000 patients

enrolled in 31 controlled trials of at least six months' duration (maximum follow-up 48 months).

Evaluation of more recent trials indicates that the advent of other preventive therapies in the years since beta-blockers were first evaluated has not attenuated the survival benefits of these drugs. Furthermore, recent experience in controlled studies has overturned the previous wisdom that beta-blockers were contraindicated in heart failure. Additional benefit may in fact be expected in this subset of MI survivors.

Beta-blockers are a pharmacologically heterogeneous group, and there are indications from meta-analyses that intrinsic sympathomimetic activity and, to a lesser extent, cardioselectivity may diminish the scale of the benefit seen in meta-analyses. Overall, it may be rational to use those individual agents that have produced the best outcomes [59].

Although not a controlled trial, the findings of the CCP are relevant to the discussion of beta-blockers post-MI. CCP investigators have reported, based on data from more than 200 000 patients, that they have found no category of post-MI patient that does not benefit from beta-blocker therapy, and that the actual benefits seen in this survey (up to 40%) were as large as or larger than those found in meta-analysis [60].

4.1.4 ACE inhibitors

Ample evidence for the benefit of ACE inhibitor therapy post-MI has emerged from controlled trials in the past decade. Distinction must be made, however, between those trials that evaluated use of ACE inhibitors early after an MI in unselected populations

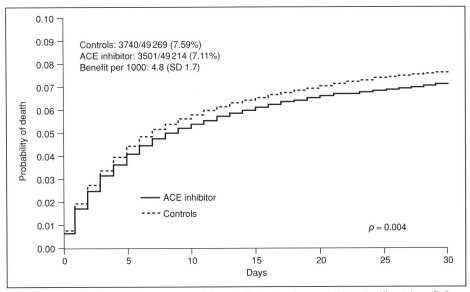

Figure 8 Effect of ACE inhibitors on post-MI mortality. There is a small but significant benefit from early use of ACE inhibitors in MI patients. The outcomes revealed in these pooled data are determined primarily by the results of the GISSI-3 and ISIS-4 clinical trials.

Reproduced with permission from ACE Inhibitor Myocardial Infarction Collaborative Group [61].

and those that examined the effects of ACE inhibition introduced later post-MI in defined higher-risk subsets.

Data for the early use of ACE inhibitors are derived from four major studies: CONSENSUS-II, GISSI-3, ISIS-4 and CCS, which collectively enrolled approximately 98 500 patients (~58 000 in ISIS-4) [61, 62]. More than 75% of patients in each study were also prescribed aspirin or other antiplatelet agents.

Pooling of data from these studies established a small but statistically significant and sustained benefit from use of ACE inhibitors early post-MI (Figure 8) [61]. This overall benefit was attributable to within-study results from GISSI-3, ISIS-4 and CCS, all of which used oral ACE inhibitor therapy. In CONSENSUS-II, parenteral administration of an ACE inhibitor was associated with an adverse outcome (net absolute risk excess ~0.9%). Within the overall data set, greater benefit was seen among higher-risk patient subgroups.

Later use of ACE inhibitors in post-MI patients has been shaped by a series of studies in patients with left ventricular dilation, a reduced ejection fraction or clinically discernible heart failure of varying degrees of severity. Pivotal studies in this arena include the AIRE study (and its extension phase, AIREX), the SAVE study and the TRACE study [63–67]. Pooled analyses of these data have confirmed a long-term survival benefit of ACE inhibitors (22% risk reduction for death) of high statistical reliability ($p < 0.001$) [67]. These data are supplemented by the findings of SOLVD, in which some two-thirds of the participating patients had a relevant history of prior MI [68, 69].

One additional recent contribution to the ACE inhibitor literature, noteworthy in the context of the reduction in sudden death with highly purified omega-3 PUFAs in GISSI-Prevenzione, is the report based on a meta-analysis that part of the overall treatment benefit with ACE inhibitors post-MI may be attributable to a 20% reduction in risk of sudden death [70].

Current guidelines for the use of ACE inhibitors endorse their early use post-MI in all patients in whom they are not contraindicated and their continued use in patients with signs or symptoms of heart failure or an ejection fraction of less than 40% and with ventricular dilation [32, 50].

4.1.5 Lipid-lowering drugs

In the context of secondary prevention, the term 'lipid-lowering drug' has been largely annexed by the statins. 4S, a large trial of several years' duration, demonstrated a 30% reduction in total mortality with simvastatin ($p = 0.0003$) in patients with a history of coronary disease and total cholesterol levels of 5.8–8.0 mmol/l [71]. Most patients (~80%) were recruited on the basis of a prior MI. Two studies with pravastatin – CARE and LIPID – have extended the benefit of statin therapy to patients with prior MI and 'average' cholesterol levels [72, 73]; the aggregate reduction in total mortality in these studies was 19% ($p < 0.0001$) [74]. Most recently, simvastatin therapy in more than 20 000 patients with established coronary disease or other high-risk characteristics was associated with a 12.9% reduction in all-cause mortality over a five-year period ($p = 0.0003$ versus placebo), and commensurate reductions in the rates of major cardiovascular events in the HPS [75].

In a meta-analysis of 28 randomized controlled trials (undertaken before publication of the HPS), statins were calculated to reduce all-cause mortality by 20% compared with all other types of lipid-lowering intervention ($p = 0.03$); none of the comparator interventions was shown to have any impact on total mortality or (with the exception of bile acid sequestrants) on any other major clinical endpoints [76].

4.1.6 Comparison of Omacor with other secondary prevention drugs

Comparison of the effects of different classes of drugs (and indeed of different drugs within any class) must be undertaken with circumspection. Differences in the circumstances of clinical trials (eg patient population studied, duration of follow-up) mean that effect sizes can vary considerably and make direct comparison across studies unreliable and potentially misleading. Reasonably informative standardized quantitative estimates can be derived, however, and when Omacor is examined in this context it is clear that the survival benefit provided by this agent compares favourably with other generally accepted types of secondary preventive therapy [77] (Table 8).

It should be recalled that use of several of these classes of drugs was widespread in the GISSI-Prevenzione study. The treatment benefit of Omacor thus appears to be additive to these other agents. Lipid-lowering drugs may be a partial exception to this statement because initial use of these drugs was low in the GISSI-Prevenzione study. Additive benefit from the combination of Omacor with statins seems probable, however, because the survival benefit of Omacor has been expressly

Intervention	Risk reduction (%)	Lives saved/1000 patient-years	NNT to save one life/year
Aspirin	16	6	~160
ACE inhibitors*	~9	4–5	~200–250
Beta-blockers	23	12	~85
Mediterranean diet**	21	6	Not available
Statins***	~20	1.6–6.2	~160–625
Omacor	20	5.7	177

Table 8 Comparison of the effects of Omacor and other recognized secondary prevention drugs on all-cause mortality post-MI.

*Results based on GISSI-3 and ISIS-4, conducted in unselected post-MI populations. Benefits of long-term ACE inhibitor therapy in post-MI patients with low left ventricular ejection fraction are consistently much larger than shown in this table.
**Based on estimates produced by the UK National Institute for Clinical Excellence (NICE) [77]. Estimates based exclusively on data from controlled trials meeting NICE criteria yield a 35% risk reduction (~18 lives saved/1000 patient-years).
***Based on interpolation of results from 4S [71], CARE [72] and LIPID [73]. Absolute and relative risk reductions and event rates varied considerably in these studies, being notably lower in CARE than in 4S or LIPID. The wide variation in outcomes is reflected in these estimates: CARE data provide the lowest number of lives saved per 1000 patient-years and the highest NNT.

dissociated from any effect on lipoprotein fractions [78] (see Chapter 5, Section 5.5).

4.1.7 Cost-effectiveness of Omacor

Any discussion of the relative cost-effectiveness of interventions needs to be undertaken with caution. First and foremost, it must be borne in mind that the results of the GISSI-Prevenzione study indicate that Omacor had a substantial clinical benefit, saving lives post-MI, notably through an effect to reduce sudden death. Furthermore, this benefit was additive to the effects of standard preventive medications. The results of cost-effectiveness studies, as with many similar analyses of other interventions, must therefore not be interpreted as a reason to favour one therapy over another. Additional benefit will be derived from using additional drugs but will incur additional costs in almost every instance. Patient benefit must be the primary consideration and the temptation to

regard health economics as a way of reducing overall health spending should be resisted.

These restrictions notwithstanding, the results of a comparison of the cost-effectiveness of Omacor and several statins indicate that the cost per life saved is likely to be well within the range currently accepted for secondary preventive therapies [79, 80]. The assessment, undertaken from a third-party perspective, was based on GISSI-Prevenzione survival data and included calculations of the incremental life-years saved by adding Omacor to standard therapy, cost of therapy, cost of hospitalization and cost of diagnostic procedures. All costs were discounted at 5% and rebased in euros (€1 = 1936.27 Italian lire). Treatment benefits were also discounted at 5%.

The discounted incremental cost of Omacor therapy during three and a half years of follow-up in the GISSI-Prevenzione study was estimated to be €817 per patient per year, a figure accounted for almost entirely by the cost of the medication itself [79]. The discounted incremental benefit of Omacor therapy during the same interval was 0.0368 life-years. The cost of Omacor therapy per life-year gained was thus €24 603 (~£15 000). Such a value would be regarded as an acceptable level of expenditure in the broader context of healthcare provision and close to being considered very favourable [80, 81]. Alternatively, based on an NNT of 177 patients treated for one year to save one life, the cost would be £31 860 per life saved (based on the current Omacor NHS price of £13.89/28 days).

5 Mechanism of Survival Benefit with Omacor

Although there is agreement about the immediate cause of the survival benefit from Omacor therapy in the GISSI-Prevenzione study – a reduction in the risk of sudden death – the mechanisms underlying this benefit have not been defined in detail.

Currently, investigators from both the GISSI-Prevenzione and the DART studies consider mechanisms related to increases in heart rate variability (HRV) and the prevention of arrhythmia and fibrillation to be likely explanations for their clinical findings with omega-3 PUFAs [23, 42]. Data from an extensive repertoire of preclinical studies and studies in humans support this hypothesis and offer insights into the possible molecular basis of these effects.

5.1 BACKGROUND ON HRV

HRV is a quantitative description of fluctuations in the interval between specified points of successive normal heartbeats. These fluctuations are regarded as representative of the state of cardiac autonomic modulation, with low HRV being indicative of (among other things) sympathetic dominance [82, 83]. A comprehensive review of the theory and practice of HRV measurement and its clinical applications has been published jointly by the Task Force of the European Society of Cardiology and the North American Society of Pacing and Electrophysiology [84]. A glossary of terms relating to HRV is given in Appendix 2.

Various methods have been developed for the measurement of HRV. One widely used method is *time-domain analysis*, of which possibly the most familiar index is SDNN, the standard deviation of all R-R intervals recorded in an electrocardiogram (ECG) recording of specified duration (often 24 hours). Other forms of time-domain analysis involve statistical comparisons of successive cardiac cycles [82]; several of these indices are believed to represent vagal regulation of the sinoatrial node.

Frequency-domain analysis is used to investigate frequency-specific oscillations in heart rate. The total amount of variance in the heart rhythm (also referred to as the power of the rhythm) is usually differentiated into four frequency bands (high, low, very low and ultra-low), each thought to be indicative of different sources of autonomic regulation [82, 83].

Nonlinear dynamics analysis is a method used for evaluating the qualitative aspects of HRV [85].

5.2 EFFECTS OF OMEGA-3 PUFAS ON HRV

5.2.1 Epidemiological observations

Low or decreased HRV has been associated with increased morbidity and mortality in numerous epidemiological studies (for a review, see Stein and Kleiger [83]) and appears to be an independent predictor of risk for sudden death and all-cause mortality in post-MI patients [84, 86]. The significance of decreased HRV as a marker of risk in MI survivors was demonstrated initially by Wolf *et al.* [87] and more recently by Kleiger and colleagues [88], who examined HRV in 808 patients an average of 11 days after an index MI. During a mean follow-up of 31 months, the relative risk of death in patients with low HRV was 5.3 times higher than that in patients with high HRV (Figure 9). Low HRV was the single strongest univariate risk factor and retained its relevance as a predictor of mortality risk after adjustment in a multivariate proportional hazards model for the effects of other Holter-documented risk factors (relative risk 2.7; chi-squared statistic [with d.f. = 1] 19.63; $p < 0.0005$) [88]. Strong adverse

correlations between low HRV and mortality post-MI have been reported more recently by the ATRAMI investigators [89].

Numerous other study groups, including the GISSI-2 investigators, have reported a strong relation between indices of decreased HRV in the early aftermath of MI and poor medium-term prognosis (for a review, see Stein and Kleiger [83]). Bigger and colleagues [90] reported correlations between frequency-domain indices (especially the very low and ultra-low power spectra) and mortality risk during four years of follow-up. This same research group has also provided evidence that decreased or low HRV up to one year after MI is predictive of

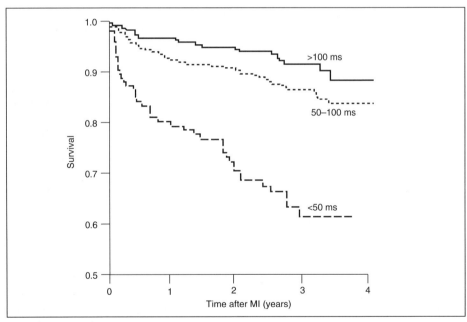

Figure 9 Association between HRV and relative risk of death in post-MI patients. Low HRV (represented by the standard deviation of all normal R-R intervals during a 24-hour period, SDNN) was associated with a markedly worse prognosis post-MI than higher HRV ($p < 0.0001$ for SDNN < 50 ms versus other groups). Data were derived from 808 patients studied on average 11 ± 3 days after an index MI.

Reproduced with permission from Kleiger *et al.* [88].

subsequent mortality [91]. An association between low HRV and clinical coronary events has also been reported in patients with stable coronary artery disease (42% of whom had had a previous MI) [92]. It is of particular relevance that decreases in HRV have been associated closely with increased risk for sudden death in many studies [93–98]. These observations impart potential clinical importance to the reports, some already discussed, of a reduction in primary cardiac arrest in individuals characterized by a high intake of omega-3 PUFAs [44, 45, 99].

5.2.2 Biochemistry studies

Studies in patients and healthy volunteers have investigated correlations between omega-3 PUFAs and HRV, and the effects of omega-3 PUFAs on arrhythmic activity. Christensen and colleagues [100, 101] reported correlations between baseline HRV and platelet fatty acid composition in 55 MI survivors enrolled in a controlled clinical trial. There was a striking correlation between platelet DHA content and HRV, with progressive increases in HRV as DHA content increased [100]. Stratification of patients by quartiles of platelet membrane DHA revealed a progressive increase in platelet EPA as DHA levels increased ($p < 0.01$ for trend), and a progressive reduction in the platelet content of arachidonic acid ($p < 0.00001$ for trend) [100].

The same investigators have since enlarged on these initial findings in two other studies in humans. In the more recent of these studies, a range of positive correlations was reported between omega-3 PUFA levels in the membranes of blood-derived cells and HRV indices in 291 patients with

suspected ischaemic coronary disease [102]. This correlation was robust in a multivariate analysis. Previously, these researchers investigated omega-3 PUFAs in cell membranes and HRV in 60 healthy volunteers and reported a linear relationship between DHA content and increased HRV [103]; this relationship was stronger in men than in women.

5.2.3 Outcome studies

There have been few direct, controlled studies of the effects of omega-3 PUFAs in humans, but the results of these studies have been consistent and indicate that omega-3 PUFAs increase HRV.

Christensen et al. demonstrated the antiarrhythmogenic potential of omega-3 PUFAs in a group of 55 MI survivors [101], reporting that 12 weeks of omega-3 PUFA supplementation was associated with a small but statistically significant increase in indices of HRV (Table 9). A similar increase in HRV indices in response to omega-3 PUFA supplementation was reported later in healthy men with initially low HRV [103]. In studies indirectly related to HRV, both Sellmayer et al. [48] and Christensen and co-workers [104] reported large and consistent reductions in VPCs in patients who received omega-3 PUFA supplementation.

These observations add to the weight of data supporting an effect of omega-3 PUFAs in preventing arrhythmias and hence sudden death. On the current balance of evidence, however, it seems likely that increased HRV is a marker for such an effect rather than part of the critical mechanism. It is conceivable that omega-3 PUFAs might increase HRV through some action to diminish the responsiveness

Treatment group	SDNN		Mean difference (95% CI)
	Before (mean ± SD)	After (mean ± SD)	
Omega-3 PUFAs	115 ± 39	124 ± 30*	+8.3 (−16 to −1)**
Controls	115 ± 45	105 ± 36	−9.4 (−2 to 20)

Table 9 Effect of omega-3 PUFA supplementation on HRV. Dietary supplementation with omega-3 PUFAs (5.2 g/day for 12 weeks) resulted in an increase in the standard deviation of all R-R intervals (SDNN, a time-domain indicator of HRV) in post-MI patients ($n = 55$) in a placebo-controlled trial.

Data from Christensen et al. [103].
*$p = 0.04$ versus baseline.
**$p = 0.01$ versus controls.

of the sinus node to incoming stimuli, but there is no direct proof of such an action. Neither is there any evidence from studies in humans that omega-3 PUFAs act centrally to influence autonomic nervous activity directly in any way that might lead to increases in HRV. Electrical effects on neurons similar to those seen in cardiomyocytes have been reported [105], however, as has an apparent anticonvulsant effect of omega-3 PUFAs in rats [106]. These data raise the fascinating possibility that electrophysiological actions of omega-3 PUFAs on the central nervous system may contribute to the prevention of cardiac arrhythmias. Considerable additional research is required, however, to test this hypothesis.

5.3 PREVENTION OF ARRHYTHMIA BY OMEGA-3 PUFAS

Pioneering investigations of the possible antiarrhythmogenic effects of omega-3 PUFAs in vivo were conducted by McLennan and colleagues in the 1980s. A clear-cut reduction in susceptibility to ventricular arrhythmias during coronary artery occlusion and reperfusion was demonstrated in rats maintained on a diet enriched with omega-3 PUFAs [107–109]. Subsequent investigations in marmosets revealed that dietary supplementation with omega-3 PUFAs for 30 months increased the threshold for the development of ventricular tachycardia in a range of situations, including acute myocardial ischaemia [110, 111]. Of note, the arrhythmia-preventing effect of omega-3 PUFAs in marmosets could not be attributed to differences in the extent of ischaemic myocardium, which was similar (~41%) in all groups, and was evident in both the presence and absence of induced myocardial ischaemia. Similarly, in rats, incidence of arrhythmias was increased in animals maintained on a diet rich in saturated fats but reduced in animals fed omega-3 PUFAs, even though there were no differences in the relative amount of ischaemic myocardium [112].

Complementary research by Billman and colleagues [113, 114] confirmed that treatment with omega-3 PUFAs prevented ischaemia-induced arrhythmias in dogs. A salient aspect of these studies was that omega-3 PUFAs were administered intravenously immediately before the induction of ischaemia (by exercise). This method of administration circumvented any possible confounding that might arise in feeding studies, enabling the investigators to conclude with a high degree of confidence that the arrhythmia-preventing effect seen in these studies was attributable to omega-3 PUFAs themselves, rather than to other materials either in the diet or produced by metabolism. In addition, Billman and colleagues [115] were satisfied that the reduction in heart rate that followed omega-3 PUFA therapy in most of their experiments was not a sufficient basis for the observed antiarrhythmogenic effects.

5.3.1 Molecular and cellular basis of arrhythmia prevention

Several mechanisms have been proposed as explanations for the observations from preclinical studies [116]. Many of the processes identified are linked closely, and it seems likely that the effects of omega-3 PUFAs are due to multiple causes rather than to any single mechanism. In broad terms, the current consensus is that omega-3 PUFAs prevent the development of arrhythmias through electrical stabilization of myocytes; effects on multiple membrane ion channels may be an integral aspect of this stabilization [117].

Although the antiarrhythmogenic effect of omega-3 PUFAs appears to be dependent on their localization within membrane phospholipids, the available evidence indicates that omega-3 PUFAs esterified in phospholipids do not exert an antiarrhythmogenic effect *per se*. For example, Weylandt *et al.* [118] studied the impact of omega-3 PUFA enrichment of membrane phospholipids in isolated rat cardiomyocytes and reported that the increased quotient of omega-3 PUFAs in membranes had no bearing on the protection provided against arrhythmogenic stimuli (isoprenaline and free calcium). Furthermore, the protective effect of omega-3 PUFAs could be abolished by pretreatment of cultures with delipidated bovine serum albumin (DBSA), which removed all unesterified omega-3 PUFAs from the cells (a finding reported earlier by Kang and Leaf [117]). These data thus indicate clearly that the antiarrhythmogenic effects of omega-3 PUFAs reside in the free fatty acids and not in the esterified forms. Such observations and conclusions are consistent with the work of Billman *et al.* [114] described already, who found that the infusion of free fatty acid forms of omega-3 PUFAs was antiarrhythmogenic in dogs. Separately, Leaf concluded that the prevention of arrhythmias by omega-3 PUFAs *in vitro* was dependent on free fatty acids partitioned into cell membranes [119].

In vitro experiments indicate that a low (<0.01) molar ratio of omega-3 PUFA to phospholipid is required in sarcolemma to achieve electrical stabilization [120]. It was concluded by these researchers that changes in the overall packing of phospholipids or a reorganization of phospholipids leading to an altered membrane fluidity could not be expected at such low concentrations. The possibility that the microenvironment of ion channels is modified by the incorporation of omega-3 PUFAs cannot, however, be excluded.

5.3.2 Electrical stabilization of cardiomyocytes and interactions with ion channels

Present thinking on the issue of omega-3 PUFAs in membrane phospholipids may be summarized in the statement that 'DHA or EPA occupying the SN2 position in phospholipids is released and protects the heart cell locally from participating in the genesis and propagation of ventricular tachycardia, which can result in cardiac arrest and sudden death. This protective effect ... depends on the unique ability of these n-3 fatty acids [omega-3 PUFAs] to stabilize all contractile heart cells electrically ...' [121].

Insights into precisely how this stabilization is achieved have been offered by studies of the effects of omega-3 PUFAs on membrane ion currents. There is an extensive literature documenting the effects of omega-3 PUFAs on ion channels and currents (see Leaf and Kang [122] for a short review). Effects have been reported on sodium, calcium and potassium currents, many of which may be pertinent to electrical stabilization and the prevention of arrhythmias.

Kang and Leaf [123] have reported distinctive effects of omega-3 PUFAs on membrane potentials in cultured neonatal rat myocytes and have concluded that omega-3 PUFAs exert protective actions on the final common pathway of arrhythmogenesis, regardless of the initiating stimulus. These protective actions involve hyperpolarization of cell membranes of ischaemic (and thus partly depolarized) cardiomyocytes, leading to prolongation of the inactivated state of the ion channels that convey the fast, voltage-dependent inward sodium current I_{Na} (Figure 10). In electrophysiological studies, exposure to omega-3 PUFAs increased the size of the electrical stimulus required to generate an action potential by some 50% and extended the effective refractory period [117, 123].

Such effects, exercised in a region of myocardial ischaemia and electrical instability, are postulated to reduce

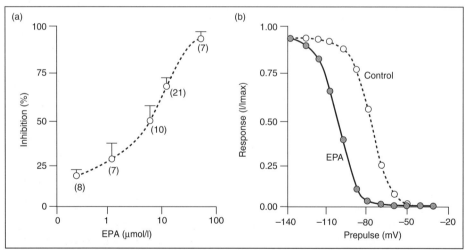

Figure 10 Effect of omega-3 PUFAs on membrane potentials. (a) Dose relation of inhibition of voltage-sensitive sodium channels by EPA. (b) EPA 10 µmol/l prolonged the inactivation state of the voltage-sensitive sodium channels, shifting the steady-state inactivation of peak sodium currents to more negative potentials.

the likelihood of arrhythmias developing [119]. All PUFAs (not only those of the omega-3 series) that have been shown to prevent arrhythmias *in vitro* affect voltage-gated sodium channels; those that do not either have no effect or are arrhythmogenic [117]. Pertinently, omega-3 PUFAs bind to the sodium channel proteins at concentrations associated with the prevention of arrhythmia [124].

A working hypothesis developed to explain these observations is that the orientation of omega-3 PUFAs within cell membranes brings the negatively charged carboxyl terminal into proximity with a positively charged region of the alpha-subunit of the ion [117, 124]. This theory reconciles the observation that prevention of arrhythmias requires *free* fatty acids; it also explains, through stereochemical considerations, why only those fatty acids that interact with the sodium channel gating complex prevent the development of arrhythmias.

The effects of omega-3 PUFAs on sodium channels have been compared with those of the class I antiarrhythmogenic drug mexiletine [125]. This comparison is pertinent to the clinical applications of the omega-3 PUFAs because mexiletine has effects on the sodium current similar to those reported with omega-3 PUFAs but, in addition, upregulates sodium channels; this upregulation is linked with an increased propensity to arrhythmias and is thought to have contributed to the unsuccessful outcome of the CAST study [19, 20]. Replication of a similar effect with omega-3 PUFAs would raise questions about the suitability of these agents for long-term clinical use.

In fact, no upregulation of sodium channels was observed in response to omega-3 PUFA treatment, a result that contrasted with the fourfold increase in numbers of sodium channels seen in response to mexiletine (Figure 11) [125]. Further investigations established that whereas mexiletine exposure was associated with a proportionate increase in levels of specific mRNA encoding the alpha-subunit of the sodium channels, no similar increase in mRNA expression occurred with omega-3 PUFAs. Both the increase in channel numbers and the enhanced expression of alpha-subunit mRNA with mexiletine could be prevented partially by the co-administration of omega-3 PUFAs.

These data have been interpreted as confirming that the arrhythmogenic potential attributed to class I antiarrhythmics on the basis of an increase in numbers of sodium channels is not shared by the omega-3 PUFAs. Furthermore, the observation that omega-3 PUFAs *prevent* the upregulation of sodium channels has been proposed as another mechanism via which these agents may prevent the development of an arrhythmogenic substrate in the ischaemic myocardium [125].

The highly conserved nature of the voltage sensor complex in mammalian sodium, potassium and calcium channels [126] means that a similar mechanism may contribute to the reported effects of omega-3 PUFAs on potassium and calcium channels. In particular, the overall electrical effect of omega-3 PUFAs on the calcium influx regulated by L-type calcium channels is qualitatively very similar to their effect on inward sodium currents [119].

Leaf and colleagues reported more than 10 years ago that omega-3 PUFAs protected isolated neonatal rat myocytes from the toxic effects of ouabain and demonstrated that this protection was due to the inhibition of the influx of ionic calcium (Figure 12a) [127, 128]. Subsequently, it was shown

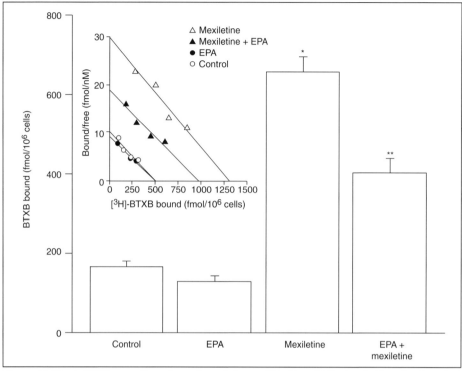

Figure 11 Effect of EPA on sodium channel regulation and binding affinity. Incubation of cultured rat cardiomyocytes with EPA 20 μM for four days had no effect on numbers of sodium channels, but EPA 20 μM significantly attenuated the increase in channel numbers seen in response to incubation with mexiletine 20 μM. Inset: the effect of EPA on sodium channel numbers in cells co-incubated with mexiletine did not include a reduction in binding affinity.

Reproduced with permission from Kang *et al.* [125].

BTXB, batrachotoxin; *$p < 0.01$ versus control; ** $p < 0.05$ versus mexiletine.

that the influx of calcium associated with ouabain use could be reproduced using the calcium channel agonist Bay K8644 and that the inhibition of that influx by omega-3 PUFAs might likewise be mimicked by the dihydropyridine calcium channel blocker nitrendipine. Both the increase in contractility seen in response to Bay K8644 and the reduction seen with nitrendipine could be prevented by co-administration of omega-3 PUFAs (EPA or DHA), effects consistent with measured changes in calcium influx [127]. In contrast to their antagonism of nitrendipine (Figure 12b), omega-3 PUFAs did not affect the reduction in contractility caused by diltiazem or verapamil. Additional analysis revealed that omega-3 PUFAs acted as noncompetitive inhibitors of specific nitrendipine binding. Numbers of both high- and low-affinity nitrendipine binding sites were reduced substantially (especially by DHA), and receptor affinity declined (Table 10) [127].

These data are compatible with omega-3 PUFAs inhibiting the influx of calcium into cells via voltage-gated L-type calcium channels, an action that

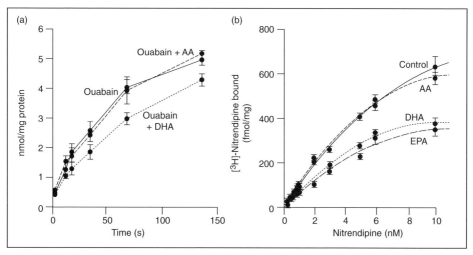

Figure 12 (a) Reduction in ouabain-induced cellular calcium overload. DHA 5 μM partly inhibited the influx of ionic calcium into cultured rat cardiomyocytes caused by treatment with ouabain 0.01 mM. Arachidonic acid (AA) 5 μM had no similar potentially protective effect. (b) Selective inhibition of nitrendipine binding to L-type calcium channels. DHA 5 μM and EPA 5 μM were non-competitive inhibitors of nitrendipine binding in isolated rat cardiomyocytes but had no similar effect on binding of verapamil or diltiazem (data not shown). These data have been interpreted as indicating that omega-3 PUFAs may modulate cellular calcium levels through effects on nitrendipine sensitive L-type calcium channels.

Reproduced with permission from Hallaq et al. [127].

Addition	High-affinity sites		Low-affinity sites	
	Affinity (K_d, nM)	Receptor numbers (fmol/mg of protein)	Affinity (K_d, nM)	Receptor numbers (fmol/mg of protein)
None	0.17±0.06	30±5	16±3	980±240
Arachidonic acid	0.18±0.08	31±4	14±4	860±150
EPA	0.005±0.0007	2.9±2	4.2±2	390±35
DHA	ND	ND	3.6±0.1	350±36

Table 10 Effect of omega-3 PUFAs on calcium channel receptors. Incubation of isolated cultured rat cardiomyocytes with EPA 5 μM or DHA 5 μM led to marked reductions in the number and affinity of specific nitrendipine receptors. In the case of DHA, suppression of high-affinity sites was so complete that binding was not detectable (ND). Arachidonic acid 5 μM had little impact on receptor-specific nitrendipine binding. Nitrendipine concentrations used in these experiments ranged from 0.03 to 10 nM.

Data from Hallaq et al. [127].

might be important for the prevention of cardiomyocyte calcium overload during ischaemia [119, 129]. The non-competitive nature of the antagonism of nitrendipine by omega-3 PUFAs suggests that the fatty acids exert this action by binding to a site functionally associated with nitrendipine receptors, rather than to the receptors themselves. Support for these conclusions is provided by the observations that, as in other studies (eg Weylandt et al. [118]), the effects of omega-3 PUFAs were abolished by pre-washing cultures with DBSA and by the finding that the effects of the beta-adrenoceptor agonist isoprenaline, which stimulates calcium influx via cardiac beta-adrenergic receptors, were not inhibited by omega-3 PUFAs [130].

It should be noted that there is no evidence that effects of omega-3 PUFAs on calcium flux have deleterious consequences for myocardial contractility or function. Recently reported observations in rat hearts *in vitro* suggest that omega-3 PUFAs are associated with lower myocardial oxygen consumption and a progressive increase in cardiac output in response to increasing workload compared with the hearts of animals maintained on a diet high in saturated fats. These data imply that omega-3 PUFA therapy is associated with enhanced myocardial efficiency and function, not a loss of contractility [131]. (In addition, hearts of PUFA-treated animals were more resistant to reperfusion arrhythmias.)

Omega-3 PUFAs have been shown to affect the function of the major cardiac voltage-dependent potassium channel (Kv1.5). In studies in Chinese hamster ovary (CHO) cells transfected with murine Kv1.5 cDNA, the addition of DHA 30 µM reduced the peak of outward potassium current and accelerated repolarization. This effect was exerted from the extracellular side of the plasma membrane, probably via a direct and highly specific action on an extracellular domain of the potassium channel [132]. (A variety of nonspecific mechanisms were excluded on the basis of experimental findings.) Additional research indicated that the attenuation of the outward rectifier potassium current was probably due to binding to the open-state channel; DHA had no effects on the inward rectifier current. Such effects could be relevant to the prevention of arrhythmias in conditions of ischaemia. A similar effect of DHA was demonstrated in isolated cultures of rat and mouse cardiomyocytes [132].

5.4 ADDITIONAL ACTIONS OF OMEGA-3 PUFAS

Omega-3 PUFAs exert a multiplicity of effects besides the increase in HRV and the prevention of arrhythmia (Figure 13) [26, 27]. Many of these other actions may be advantageous in patients with ischaemic heart disease, although some current interpretations of the evidence assign these actions a role ancillary to the central mechanism of arrhythmia prevention. In several instances, most of these effects have been reported with higher doses than are needed to prevent arrhythmias.

5.4.1 Limitation of infarct size

Singh et al. [133] have reported a reduction in infarct size (determined by indirect methods) in patients treated with omega-3 PUFAs (EPA 1 g/day)

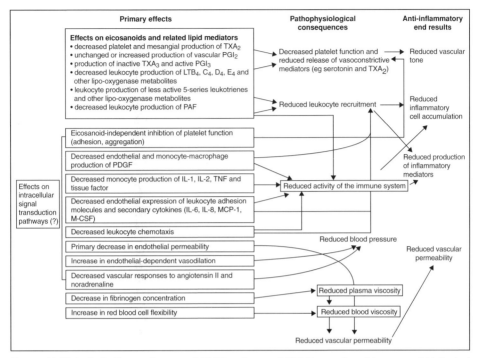

Figure 13 Biological effects of omega-3 PUFAs. Omega-3 PUFAs exert a wide range of biological effects that may be relevant to the prevention of atherosclerosis, especially when used at high dosage.

Reproduced with permission from De Caterina *et al.* [27].

and have suggested that this effect contributes to reduced MI-related mortality. However, infarct size also influences the electrical stability of the heart, and a parallel reduction in the proportion of patients developing arrhythmias was observed in this study. It is thus difficult to differentiate indirect benefits in suppression of arrhythmia arising from reductions in infarct size from a more direct inhibition of arrhythmia. From a practical point of view, it needs to be recognized that in situations where thrombolytic therapy is routine, any contribution from omega-3 PUFAs to the limitation of infarct size is likely to be small and of uncertain clinical relevance.

5.4.2 Effects on the arachidonic acid cascade and atherosclerosis

An extensive range of antiplatelet and anti-inflammatory effects has been attributed to PUFAs as a result of reduced production of arachidonate-derived prostanoids and the physiological antagonism of those compounds [27]. The basis for these effects is competitive substitution of omega-3 PUFAs (especially EPA) for arachidonic acid in the cyclo-oxygenase and lipo-oxygenase pathways, with both quantitative and qualitative consequences (Figure 14). The quantity of metabolites is reduced (because omega-3 PUFAs are less satisfactory enzyme substrates than is arachidonic acid), and metabolism is diverted toward less physiologically active forms of prostanoids and leukotrienes than are derived from arachidonate. In particular, production of thromboxane A_2 is restricted in favour of the markedly less pro-aggregatory thromboxane A_3 (Figure 14) [26].

The overall balance of activity resulting from these changes disposes toward vasodilation and the inhibition of platelet aggregation and away from vasoconstriction and thrombus formation. Parallel shifts in the synthesis of cytokines are inferred to result in a shift to a less inflammatory *milieu* and hence to a reduced potential for the development of atherosclerotic lesions [27, 134–136].

Reductions in levels of platelet-derived growth factors and macrophage chemoattractant protein might also be expected to inhibit the progress of atherosclerosis [137].

There are reasons for believing, however, that in addition to these longer-term antiatherosclerotic effects, a measure of the benefit obtained by disrupting the arachidonic acid cascade with omega-3 PUFAs can be traced back to the arrhythmia-preventing qualities of these compounds. First, it should be noted that the arachidonic acid cascade is initiated by release of the free acid form from the SN2 position in membrane phospholipids. Omega-3 PUFAs are able to engage in substrate inhibition of arachidonate

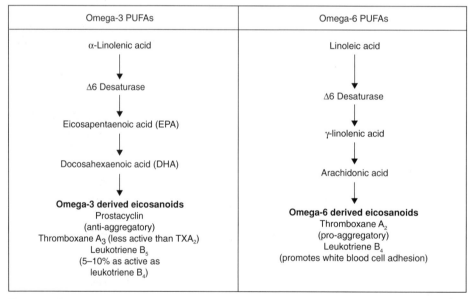

Figure 14 Omega-3 PUFAs and arachidonic acid pathways. The pathways have several enzymes in common. Omega-3 PUFAs are therefore able to inhibit the synthesis of arachidonic acid. In addition, the products of omega-3 PUFA metabolism are less atherogenic and pro-aggregatory than many arachidonic acid derivatives. (Note: the linear progress from EPA to DHA represents the major metabolic pathway. However, retroconversion of DHA to EPA can occur.)

metabolism when they substitute for arachidonic acid at the SN2 site. The importance of omega-3 PUFAs released from this site in the electrical stabilization of cardiomyocytes has already been discussed. In addition, both arachidonic acid and thromboxane A_2 have been reported to have arrhythmogenic qualities [117, 138].

5.4.3 Inhibition of thrombus formation

Multiple effects of omega-3 PUFAs on platelet function and blood clotting have been described, including reductions in platelet count and augmentation of fibrinolytic activity (Table 11) [26, 139–141]. These effects could be expected to reduce the potential for thrombus (or embolus) formation in the vicinity of a ruptured atherosclerotic plaque, so reducing the risk of a clinical ischaemic event.

A reduction in plasminogen activator inhibitor 1 (PAI-1) levels has been reported in response to omega-3 PUFA supplementation in patients with established coronary disease, with no corresponding reduction in the activity of tissue plasminogen activator [139]. Such an effect might be expected to reduce the tendency to thrombus formation. This effect was seen with much higher doses of omega-3 PUFAs than were evaluated in the GISSI-Prevenzione study, however, so the relevance of this report to the results of GISSI-Prevenzione is uncertain.

Clinical evidence for a modest inhibition of atherosclerosis progression by omega-3 PUFAs has been obtained in at least one angiography study [142]. Data relating to restenosis, a physiologically distinct entity from primary atherosclerosis, are inconsistent [143, 144], although the report that DHA induces apoptosis in vascular smooth muscle cells *in vitro* would seem to be compatible with an anti-restenosis potential [145].

Factor	Role in atherosclerosis	Effect of omega-3 PUFAs on factor concentration
Arachidonic acid	Thromboxane and leukotriene precursor	Decreased
Thromboxane A_2	Platelet aggregation; vasoconstriction	Decreased
Fibrinogen	Promotes blood clotting	Decreased
Platelet-activating factor	Platelet activation	Decreased
Plasminogen activator inhibitor 1	Promotes blood clotting	Decreased
Platelet-derived growth factor	Chemoattractant and mitogen for macrophages and vascular smooth muscle cells	Decreased
Tissue plasminogen activator	Increased fibrinolysis	Increased

Table 11 Effect of omega-3 PUFAs on platelet function and blood clotting. Omega-3 PUFAs exert favourable effects on levels of numerous factors implicated in atherogenesis or the progression of atherosclerosis, with a presumed net antiatherosclerotic action.

Data from Harper and Jacobson [26] and Mehta et al. [139].

5.5 LIPID CHANGES UNLIKELY TO BE INVOLVED IN PREVENTION OF SUDDEN DEATH

One mechanism that may be excluded with a degree of confidence is an effect mediated via lipids [78]. Changes in lipoprotein and triglyceride fractions in patients randomized to Omacor at the dose of 1 g/day used in the GISSI-Prevenzione study were small; levels of LDL cholesterol, the principal lipid-related risk determinant of atherosclerotic coronary disease, rose slightly and not significantly. Such effects seen in conjunction with large and statistically significant improvements in survival are incompatible with the cholesterol hypothesis of atherosclerosis and with experience in a multiplicity of large, rigorously controlled trials of lipid-lowering agents. In this context, it should be recalled that a substantial proportion of the patients in the GISSI-Prevenzione study (more than 40% in the later stages of enrolment) were receiving statin therapy: the clinical impact of Omacor was additional to any benefit from these drugs and, by inference from the average lipoprotein changes, exerted through some other mechanism. Moreover, the time course of benefit in the GISSI-Prevenzione study, with a reduction in all-cause mortality in the first three months and in several forms of cause-specific mortality within six months, differs from that seen in trials of lipid-lowering drugs, in which conclusive treatment benefits took 12 months or more to emerge (eg see Scandinavian Simvastatin Survival Study Group [71] and Heart Protection Study Collaborative Group [75]).

The conclusion that lipid-related effects made no substantive contribution to the clinical benefits of Omacor therapy in the GISSI-Prevenzione study extends to effects on triglycerides. The triglyceride-lowering effect reported with high doses of Omacor ($\geqslant$4 g/day) [146, 147] was not replicated in the GISSI-Prevenzione study and there is no reason to believe that the less than 5% reduction in triglyceride levels seen in the study had any bearing on the clinical outcomes reported. A similar phenomenon of clinical benefit despite notionally unfavourable changes in lipoprotein levels has been reported in a separate controlled trial of omega-3 PUFA therapy [142].

6 Conclusions

A wealth of evidence from laboratory research, through epidemiological and clinical studies to randomized clinical trials, indicates that omega-3 PUFAs have a relevant role in cardiovascular disease.

The GISSI-Prevenzione study was designed to transform routine clinical activity into an experimental exercise within the framework of a cooperative, public health-oriented network of clinical cardiologists. The significant reduction in total mortality obtained with Omacor treatment during the trial was confirmation, in a prospective investigation of observations in a series of large cohort studies, and a corroboration, in a substantially larger patient population, of the results of DART, a randomized controlled trial. That improvement in overall survival was underwritten by a significant and impressive reduction in sudden death, which seems to be due to the antiarrhythmogenic effect of omega-3 PUFAs observed by Alexander Leaf and Peter McLennan in their studies on cultured myocytes, rats, dogs and marmosets.

Such an antiarrhythmic effect, although at variance with the expectations generated from observations of antiatherosclerotic, anti-inflammatory and anti-thrombotic effects of omega-3 PUFAs (documented before and during the GISSI-Prevenzione study), integrates well with the mechanisms of action and clinical benefit of antiplatelet agents, beta-blockers, ACE inhibitors and statins, all of which were represented amply in GISSI-Prevenzione. Indeed, the benefits of Omacor were obtained in a large population of post-MI patients with relatively well preserved left ventricular function, with broadly correct dietary habits, and receiving up-to-date pharmacological preventive interventions. This potential antiarrhythmogenic action provides a rationale for the use of Omacor in the management of post-MI patients.

The results of the GISSI-Prevenzione study introduce Omacor, used at a dose virtually devoid of a cholesterol-lowering effect, into a post-MI scientific scenario dominated largely by the cholesterol–heart hypothesis. This divergence should be regarded, however, as a matter of interest and a spur to further clinical research rather than as a problem or a discrepancy to be explained away or ignored. Indeed, the experience of the GISSI-Prevenzione trial – including the documentation of a very good safety and tolerability record for low-dose Omacor – suggests applications for this therapeutic principle beyond the post-MI population.

Two populations in particular may offer further opportunities to test the clinical and epidemiological relevance of Omacor:

- Patients who have not yet suffered a cardiovascular event, ie people who are usually classified as candidates for primary prevention strategies.
- Patients at the other extreme of the spectrum of morbidity from primary prevention, namely those who have developed heart failure and who often still have a poor short- to medium-term prognosis

despite the impressive therapeutic advances of the last decade.

The possibility of replicating the findings of the GISSI-Prevenzione study, especially the reduction in sudden death, in these populations is an immensely exciting prospect.

A note of caution and encouragement is needed at this point. GISSI-Prevenzione established Omacor, used at low doses, as a valid and valuable pharmacological intervention post-MI. It can be anticipated, however, that an emphasis on dietary modifications may be considered an effective alternative to this therapy. It is important that time and resources are devoted to dismantling this conceptual barrier: it is clear from the results of GISSI-Prevenzione that whatever exertions may be made in improving dietary habits, the use of Omacor provides important additional clinical benefits. Dietary advice and PUFA supplementation are complementary parts of a treatment strategy, not mutually exclusive choices. This message needs to be conveyed clearly to patients and physicians alike.

Roberto Marchioli, MD
Head, Laboratory of Clinical
Epidemiology of Cardiovascular Disease
Consorzio Mario Negri Sud
Santa Maria Imbaro, Italy

Appendix 1   Study Acronyms

AIRE	Acute Infarction Ramipril Efficacy	HOPE	Heart Outcomes Prevention Evaluation
AIREX	AIRE Extension	HOT	Hypertension Optimal Treatment
ATBC	Alpha-Tocopherol, Beta-Carotene Cancer Prevention Study	HPS	Heart Protection Study
		ISIS	International Study of Infarct Survival
ATRAMI	Autonomic Tone and Reflexes After Myocardial Infarction	LIPID	Long-term Intervention with Pravastatin in Ischaemic Disease
AVID	Antiarrhythmics Versus Implantable Defibrillators	MADIT	Multicenter Automatic Defibrillator Implantation Trial
CARE	Cholesterol and Recurrent Events	MUSTT	Multicenter Unsustained Tachycardia Trial
CASH	Cardiac Arrest Study Hamburg	4S	Scandinavian Simvastatin Survival Study
CAST	Cardiac Arrhythmia Suppression Trial		
CCP	Cooperative Cardiovascular Project	SAVE	Survival and Ventricular Enlargement
CCS	Chinese Cardiac Study	SCD-HeFT	Sudden Cardiac Death in Heart Failure Trial
CHAOS	Cambridge Heart Antioxidant Study		
CIDS	Canadian Implantable Defibrillator Study	SOLVD	Studies of Left Ventricular Dysfunction
CONSENSUS-II	Cooperative New Scandinavian Enalapril Survival Study	SPACE	Secondary Prevention with Antioxidants of Cardiovascular Disease in End-stage Renal Disease
DART	Diet and Re-infarction Trial		
GISSI	Gruppo Italiano per lo Studio della Sopravvivenza nell'Infarto Miocardico	TRACE	Trandolapril Cardiac Evaluation

Appendix 2 Glossary of Heart Rate Variability Terms

TIME-DOMAIN INDICES OF HEART RATE VARIABILITY

Variable	Unit	Definition
SDNN	Milliseconds	Standard deviation of all normal R-R intervals in a 24-hour ECG
SDANN	Milliseconds	Standard deviation of the mean of all five-minute segments of normal R-R intervals in a 24-hour ECG
SDNNIDX	Milliseconds	Mean of the standard deviations of all normal R-R intervals of all five-minute segments in a 24-hour ECG
pNN50	Per cent	Percentage difference between adjacent normal R-R intervals > 50 ms in an entire 24-hour ECG
r-MSSD	Milliseconds	Root mean square successive differences: the square root of the mean of the sum of the squares of differences between adjacent normal R-R intervals in an entire 24-hour ECG
Baseline width	Milliseconds	Width of baseline of main triangle superimposed on the histogram of R-R intervals

FREQUENCY-DOMAIN INDICES OF HEART RATE VARIABILITY

Variable	Frequency range (Hz)	Cycles/unit time
High-frequency power	0.15–0.40	9–24/min
Low-frequency power	0.04–0.15	2.4–9/min
Very low-frequency power	0.0033–0.04	0.2–2.4/min
Ultra-low-frequency power	1.15×10^{-5}–0.0033	1/24 h–0.2/min
Total power	$1.15 \times 10^{-5} \times 0.40$	1/24 h–24/min

References

1. Braunwald E. Evolution of the management of acute myocardial infarction: a 20th century saga. *Lancet* 1998; **352**: 1771–4.
2. McGovern PG, Jacobs DR, Shahar E *et al*. Trends in acute coronary heart disease mortality, morbidity, and medical care from 1985 through 1997. The Minnesota Heart Survey. *Circulation* 2001; **104**: 19–24.
3. Abrahamsson P, Dellborg M, Rosengren A *et al*. Improved long term prognosis after myocardial infarction 1984–1991. *Eur Heart J* 1998; **19**: 1512–17.
4. McGovern PG, Pankow JS, Shahar E *et al*. Recent trends in acute coronary heart disease. Mortality, morbidity, medical care, and risk factors. *N Engl J Med* 1996; **334**: 884–90.
5. Stewart AW, Beaglehole R, Jackson R, Bingley W. Trends in three-year survival following acute myocardial infarction, 1983–1992. *Eur Heart J* 1999; **20**: 803–7.
6. Capewell S, Livingston BM, MacIntyre K *et al*. Trends in case-fatality in 117 718 patients admitted with acute myocardial infarction in Scotland. *Eur Heart J* 2000; **21**: 1833–40.
7. Haffner SM, Lehto S, Rönnemaa T *et al*. Mortality from coronary heart disease in subjects with type 2 diabetes and in nondiabetic subjects with and without prior myocardial infarction. *N Engl J Med* 1998; **339**: 229–34.
8. Lampe FC, Whincup PH, Wannamethee SG *et al*. The natural history of prevalent ischaemic heart disease in middle-aged men. *Eur Heart J* 2000; **21**: 1052–62.
9. ASPIRE Steering Group. A British Cardiac Society survey of the potential for the secondary prevention of coronary disease: ASPIRE (Action on Secondary Prevention through Intervention to Reduce Events) principal results. *Heart* 1996; **75**: 334–42.
10. EUROASPIRE Study Group. A European Society of Cardiology survey of secondary prevention of coronary heart disease: principal results. *Eur Heart J* 1997; **18**: 1569–82.
11. De Lorgeril M, Salen P. Diet as preventive medicine in cardiology. *Curr Opin Cardiol* 2000; **15**: 364–70.
12. Priori SG, Aliot E, Blomstrom-Lundqvist C *et al*. Task Force on Sudden Cardiac Death of the European Society of Cardiology. *Eur Heart J* 2001; **22**: 1374–450.
13. Huikuri HV, Castellanos A, Myerburg RJ. Sudden death due to cardiac arrhythmias. *N Engl J Med* 2001; **345**: 1473–81.
14. Myerburg RJ, Spooner PM. Opportunities for sudden death prevention: directions for new clinical and basic research. *Cardiovasc Res* 2001; **50**: 177–85.
15. Myerburg RJ, Mitrani R, Interian A Jr, Castellanos A. Interpretation of outcomes of antiarrhythmic clinical trials. Design features and population impact. *Circulation* 1998; **97**: 1514–21.
16. The Antiarrhythmics versus Implantable Defibrillators (AVID) Investigators. A comparison of antiarrhythmic-drug therapy with implantable defibrillators in patients resuscitated from near-fatal ventricular arrhythmias. *N Engl J Med* 1997; **337**: 1576–83.
17. Moss AJ, Hall WJ, Cannom DS *et al*. Improved survival with an implanted defibrillator in patients with coronary disease at high risk for ventricular arrhythmia. *N Engl J Med* 1996; **335**: 1933–40.
18. Coletta A, Thackray S, Nikitin N, Cleland JGF. Clinical trials update: highlights of the scientific sessions of the

American College of Cardiology 2002: LIFE, DANAMI 2, MADIT-2, MIRACLE-ICD, OVERTURE, OCTAVE, ENABLE 1 & 2, CHRISTMAS, AFFIRM, RACE, WIZARD, AZACS, REMATCH, BNP trial and HARDBALL. *Eur J Heart Fail* 2002; **4**: 381–8.

19. Echt DS, Liebson PR, Mitchell LB *et al*. Mortality and morbidity in patients receiving encainide, flecainide, or placebo. The Cardiac Arrhythmia Suppression Trial. *N Engl J Med* 1991; **324**: 781–8.

20. The Cardiac Arrhythmia Suppression Trial II Investigators. Effect of the antiarrhythmic agent moricizine on survival after myocardial infarction. *N Engl J Med* 1992; **327**: 227–33.

21. Siebels J, Cappato R, Rüppel R *et al*. Preliminary results of the Cardiac Arrest Study Hamburg (CASH). *Am J Cardiol* 1993; **72**: 109F–13F.

22. GISSI-Prevenzione Investigators. Dietary supplementation with n-3 polyunsaturated fatty acids and vitamin E after myocardial infarction: results of the GISSI-Prevenzione trial. *Lancet* 1999; **354**: 447–55.

23. Marchioli R, Barzi F, Bomba E *et al*. Early protection against sudden death by n-3 polyunsaturated fatty acids after myocardial infarction. Time-course analysis of the results of Gruppo Italiano per lo Studio della Sopravvivenza nell'Infarto Miocardico (GISSI)-Prevenzione. *Circulation* 2002; **105**: 1897–903.

24. Marchioli R, on behalf of the GISSI-Prevenzione Investigators. Treatment with n-3 polyunsaturated fatty acids after myocardial infarction: results of GISSI-Prevenzione Trial. *Eur Heart J Suppl* 2001; **3(suppl D)**: 85–97.

25. Omacor SmPC, Solvay Pharmaceuticals GmBH. Available in the online *Electronic Medicines Compendium* (http://emc.vhn.net).

26. Harper CR, Jacobson TA. The fats of life. The role of omega-3 fatty acids in the prevention of coronary heart disease. *Arch Intern Med* 2001; **161**: 2185–92.

27. De Caterina R, Basta G. n-3 Fatty acids and the inflammatory response – biological background. *Eur Heart J Suppl* 2001; **3(suppl D)**: 42–9.

28. Rupp H, Turcani M, Ohkubo T *et al*. Dietary linolenic acid-mediated increase in vascular prostacyclin formation. *Mol Cell Biochem* 1996; **162**: 59–64.

29. Ohkubo T, Jacob R, Rupp H. Swimming changes vascular fatty acid composition and prostanoid generation of rats. *Am J Physiol* 1992; **262**: R464–71.

30. Grynberg A, Ziegler D, Rupp H. Sympathoadrenergic overactivity and lipid metabolism. *Cardiovasc Drugs Ther* 1996; **10**: 223–30.

31. Hansson L, Zanchetti A, Carruthers SG *et al*. Effects of intensive blood-pressure lowering and low-dose aspirin in patients with hypertension: principal results of the Hypertension Optimal Treatment (HOT) randomised trial. *Lancet* 1998; **351**: 1755–62.

32. Wood D, de Backer, Faergeman O *et al*. Prevention of coronary heart disease in clinical practice. Recommendations of the Second Joint Task Force of European and other Societies on Coronary Prevention. *Eur Heart J* 1998; **19**: 1434–503.

33. Violi F, Micheletta F, Iuliano L. Antioxidants and atherosclerosis. *Eur Heart J Suppl* 2002; **4(suppl B)**: B17–21.

34. Jha P, Flather M, Lonn E *et al*. The antioxidant vitamins and cardiovascular disease. A critical review of epidemiologic and clinical trial data. *Ann Intern Med* 1995; **123**: 860–72.

35. Heart Outcomes Prevention Evaluation Study Investigators. Vitamin E supplementation and cardiovascular events in high-risk patients. *N Engl J Med* 2000; **342**: 154–60.

36. Heart Protection Study Collaborative Group. MRC/BHF Heart Protection Study of antioxidant vitamin supplementation in 20 536 high-risk individuals: a randomised placebo-controlled trial. *Lancet* 2002; **360**: 23–33.

37. Pietinen P, Ascherio A, Korhonen P et al. Intake of fatty acids and risk of coronary heart disease in a cohort of Finnish men. The Alpha-Tocopherol, Beta-Carotene Cancer Prevention Study. Am J Epidemiol 1997; **145**: 876–87.

38. Boaz M, Smetana S, Weinstein T et al. Secondary prevention with antioxidants of cardiovascular disease in endstage renal disease (SPACE): randomised placebo-controlled trial. Lancet 2000; **356**: 1213–18.

39. Stephens NG, Parsons A, Schofield PM et al. Randomised controlled trial of vitamin E in patients with coronary disease: Cambridge Heart Antioxidant Study (CHAOS). Lancet 1996; **347**: 781–6.

40. Meagher EA, Barry OP, Lawson JA et al. Effects of vitamin E on lipid peroxidation in healthy persons. JAMA 2001; **285**: 1178–82.

41. Burr ML, Fehily AM, Gilbert JF et al. Effects of changes in fat, fish, and fibre intakes on death and myocardial reinfarction: Diet and Reinfarction Trial (DART). Lancet 1989; **2**: 757–61.

42. Burr ML. Reflections on the Diet and Reinfarction Trial (DART). Eur Heart J Suppl 2001; **3(suppl D)**: D75–8.

43. De Lorgeril M, Salen P, Defaye P et al. Dietary prevention of sudden cardiac death. Eur Heart J 2002; **23**: 277–85.

44. Albert CM, Campos H, Stampfer MJ et al. Blood levels of long-chain n-3 fatty acids and the risk of sudden death. N Engl J Med 2002; **346**: 1113–18.

45. Siscovick DS, Raghunathan TE, King I et al. Dietary intake and cell membrane levels of long-chain n-3 polyunsaturated fatty acids and the risk of primary cardiac arrest. JAMA 1995; **274**: 1363–7.

46. Maggioni AP, Tavazzi L, Marchioli R et al. Perspectives on n-3 PUFAs: primary prevention, antiarrhythmic effects, congestive heart failure. Eur Heart J Suppl 2001; **3(suppl D)**: D106–9.

47. Hu FB, Bronner L, Willett WC et al. Fish and omega-3 fatty acid intake and risk of coronary heart disease in women. JAMA 2002; **287**: 1815–21.

48. Sellmayer A, Witzgall H, Lorenz RL, Weber PC. Effects of dietary fish oil on ventricular premature complexes. Am J Cardiol 1995; **76**: 974–7.

49. Smith SC, Blair SN, Criqui MH et al. Preventing heart attack and death in patients with coronary disease. J Am Coll Cardiol 1995; **26**: 292–4.

50. Smith SC, Blair SN, Bonow RO et al. AHA/ACC guidelines for preventing heart attack and death in patients with atherosclerotic cardiovascular disease: 2001 update. A statement for healthcare professionals from the American Heart Association and the American College of Cardiology. Circulation 2001; **104**: 1577–9.

51. Fibrinolytic Therapy Trialists' (FTT) Collaborative Group. Indications for fibrinolytic therapy in suspected acute myocardial infarction: collaborative overview of early mortality and major morbidity results from all randomised trials of more than 1000 patients. Lancet 1994; **343**: 311–22.

52. Elwood PC, Cochrane AL, Burr ML et al. A randomized controlled trial of acetyl salicylic acid in the secondary prevention of mortality from myocardial infarction. BMJ 1974; **1**: 436–40.

53. Boston Collaborative Drug Surveillance Group. Regular aspirin intake and acute myocardial infarction. BMJ 1974; **1**: 440–43.

54. Antiplatelet Trialists' Collaboration. Collaborative overview of randomised trials of antiplatelet therapy – I: prevention of death, myocardial infarction, and stroke by prolonged antiplatelet therapy in various categories of patients. BMJ 1994; **308**: 81–106.

55. Antithrombotic Trialists' Collaboration. Collaborative meta-analysis of randomised trials of antiplatelet therapy for prevention of death, myocardial infarction, and stroke in high risk patients. BMJ 2002; **324**: 71–86.

56. Anand SS, Yusuf S. Oral anticoagulant therapy in patients with coronary artery disease: a meta-analysis. *JAMA* 1999; **282**: 2058–67.

57. Mehta RH, Eagle KA. Secondary prevention in acute myocardial infarction. *BMJ* 1998; **316**: 838–42.

58. Freemantle N, Cleland J, Young P *et al*. Beta blockade after myocardial infarction: systematic review and meta regression analysis. *BMJ* 1999; **318**: 1730–37.

59. Shivkumar K. Long-term β-blocker use reduces mortality after myocardial infarction (commentary). *Evidence-Based Med* 2000; **5**: 12.

60. Gottlieb SS, McCarter RJ, Vogel RA. Effect of beta-blockade on mortality among high-risk and low-risk patients after myocardial infarction. *N Engl J Med* 1998; **339**: 489–97.

61. ACE Inhibitor Myocardial Infarction Collaborative Group. Indications for ACE inhibitors in the early treatment of acute myocardial infarction. Systematic overview of individual data from 100 000 patients in randomized trials. *Circulation* 1998; **97**: 2202–12.

62. Latini R, Maggioni AP, Flather M *et al*. ACE inhibitor use in patients with myocardial infarction. Summary of evidence from clinical trials. *Circulation* 1995; **92**: 3132–7.

63. Hall AS, Murray GD, Ball SG *et al*. Follow-up study of patients randomly allocated ramipril or placebo for heart failure after acute myocardial infarction: AIRE Extension (AIREX) Study. *Lancet* 1997; **349**: 1493–7.

64. Pfeffer MA, Braunwald E, Moyé LA *et al*. Effect of captopril on mortality and morbidity in patients with left ventricular dysfunction after myocardial infarction. Results of the Survival and Ventricular Enlargement trial. *N Engl J Med* 1992; **327**: 669–77.

65. The Acute Infarction Ramipril Efficacy (AIRE) Study Investigators. Effect of ramipril on mortality and morbidity of survivors of acute myocardial infarction with clinical evidence of heart failure. *Lancet* 1993; **342**: 821–8.

66. Køber L, Torp-Pedersen C, Carlsen JE *et al*. A clinical trial of the angiotensin-converting-enzyme inhibitor trandolapril in patients with left ventricular dysfunction after myocardial infarction. *N Engl J Med* 1995; **333**: 1670–76.

67. Hennekens CH, Albert CM, Godfried SL *et al*. Adjunctive drug therapy of acute myocardial infarction – evidence from clinical trials. *N Engl J Med* 1996; **335**: 1660–67.

68. The SOLVD Investigators. Effect of enalapril on survival in patients with reduced left ventricular ejection fractions and congestive heart failure. *N Engl J Med* 1991; **325**: 293–302.

69. The SOLVD Investigators. Effect of enalapril on mortality and the development of heart failure in asymptomatic patients with reduced left ventricular ejection fractions. *N Engl J Med* 1992; **327**: 685–91.

70. Domanski MJ, Exner DV, Borkowf CB *et al*. Effect of angiotensin converting enzyme inhibition on sudden cardiac death in patients following acute myocardial infarction. A meta-analysis of randomized clinical trials. *J Am Coll Cardiol* 1999; **33**: 598–604.

71. Scandinavian Simvastatin Survival Study Group. Randomised trial of cholesterol lowering in 4444 patients with coronary heart disease: the Scandinavian Simvastatin Survival Study (4S). *Lancet* 1994; **344**: 1383–9.

72. Sacks FM, Pfeffer MA, Moye LA *et al*. The effect of pravastatin on coronary events after myocardial infarction in patients with average cholesterol levels. *N Engl J Med* 1996; **335**: 1001–9.

73. The Long-term Intervention with Pravastatin in Ischaemic Disease (LIPID) Study Group. Prevention of cardiovascular events and death with pravastatin in patients with coronary heart disease and a broad range of initial cholesterol levels. *N Engl J Med* 1998; **339**: 1349–57.

74. Simes J, Furberg CD, Braunwald E et al. Effects of pravastatin on mortality in patients with and without coronary heart disease across a broad range of cholesterol levels. Eur Heart J 2002; 23: 207–15.

75. Heart Protection Study Collaborative Group. MRC/BHF Heart Protection Study of cholesterol lowering with simvastatin in 20 536 high-risk individuals: a randomised placebo-controlled trial. Lancet 2002; 360: 7–22.

76. Bucher HC, Griffith LE, Guyatt GH. Effect of HMGCoA reductase inhibitors on stroke. A meta-analysis of randomized, controlled trials. Ann Intern Med 1998; 128: 89–95.

77. www.nice.org.uk (accessed 11 September 2002).

78. Marchioli R, Valagussa F on behalf of GISSI-Prevenzione Investigators. The results of the GISSI-Prevenzione trial in the general framework of secondary prevention. Eur Heart J 2000; 21: 949–52.

79. Franzosi MG, Brunetti M, Marchioli R et al. Cost-effectiveness analysis of n-3 polyunsaturated fatty acids (PUFA) after myocardial infarction. Pharmacoeconomics 2001; 19: 411–20.

80. Tengs TO, Adams ME, Pliskin JS et al. Five-hundred life-saving interventions and their cost-effectiveness. Risk Anal 1995; 15: 369–90.

81. Boriani G, Biffi M, Martignani C et al. Cost-effectiveness of implantable cardioverter-defibrillators. Eur Heart J 2001; 22: 990–96.

82. Stein PK, Bosner MS, Kleiger RE, Conger BM. Heart rate variability: a measure of cardiac autonomic tone. Am Heart J 1994; 127: 1376–81.

83. Stein PK, Kleiger RE. Insights from the study of heart rate variability. Annu Rev Med 1999; 50: 249–61.

84. Task Force of the European Society of Cardiology and the North American Society of Pacing Electrophysiology. Heart rate variability. Standards of measurement, physiological interpretation, and clinical use. Circulation 1996; 93: 1043–65.

85. Lombardi F, Mäkikallio TH, Myerburg RJ, Huikuri HV. Sudden cardiac death: role of heart rate variability to identify patients at risk. Cardiovasc Res 2001; 50: 210–17.

86. Van Ravenswaaij-Arts CMA, Kollée LAA, Hopman JCW et al. Heart rate variability. Ann Intern Med 1993; 118: 436–47.

87. Wolf MM, Varigos GA, Hunt D, Sloman JG. Sinus arrhythmia in acute myocardial infarction. Med J Aust 1978; 2: 52–3.

88. Kleiger RE, Miller JP, Bigger JT et al. Decreased heart rate variability and its association with increased mortality after acute myocardial infarction. Am J Cardiol 1987; 59: 256–62.

89. La Rovere MT, Bigger JT Jr, Marcus FI et al. Baroreflex sensitivity and heart-rate variability in prediction of total cardiac mortality after myocardial infarction. Lancet 1998; 351: 478–84.

90. Bigger JT, Fleiss JL, Steinman RC et al. Frequency domain measures of heart period variability and mortality after myocardial infarction. Circulation 1992; 85: 164–71.

91. Bigger JT, Fleiss JL, Rolnitzky LM, Steinman RC. Frequency domain measures of heart period variability to assess risk late after myocardial infarction. J Am Coll Cardiol 1993; 21: 729–36.

92. Van Boven AJ, Jukema JW, Haaksma J et al. Depressed heart rate variability is associated with events in patients with stable coronary artery disease and preserved left ventricular function. Am Heart J 1998; 135: 571–6.

93. Hartikainen JEK, Malik M, Staunton A et al. Distinction between arrhythmic and nonarrhythmic death after acute myocardial infarction based on heart rate variability, signal-averaged electrocardiogram, ventricular arrhythmias and left ventricular ejection fraction. J Am Coll Cardiol 1996; 28: 296–304.

94. Algra A, Tijssen JGP, Roelandt JRTC et al. Heart rate variability from 24-hour electrocardiography and the 2-year risk for sudden death. *Circulation* 1993; **88**: 180–85.

95. Mølgaard H, Sørensen KE, Bjerregaard P. Attenuated 24-h heart rate variability in apparently healthy subjects, subsequently suffering sudden cardiac death. *Clin Auton Res* 1991; **1**: 233–7.

96. Myers GA, Martin GJ, Magid NM et al. Power spectral analysis of heart rate variability in sudden cardiac death: comparison to other methods. *IEEE Trans Biomed Eng* 1986; **33**: 1149–56.

97. Martin GJ, Magid NM, Myers G et al. Heart rate variability and sudden death secondary to coronary artery disease during ambulatory electrocardiographic monitoring. *Am J Cardiol* 1987; **60**: 86–9.

98. Nakagawa M, Saikawa T, Ito M. Progressive reduction of heart rate variability with eventual sudden death in two patients. *Br Heart J* 1994; **71**: 87–8.

99. Albert CM, Hennekens CH, O'Donnell CJ et al. Fish consumption and risk of sudden cardiac death. *JAMA* 1998; **279**: 23–8.

100. Christensen JH, Korup E, Aarøe J et al. Fish consumption, n-3 fatty acids in cell membranes, and heart rate variability in survivors of myocardial infarction with left ventricular dysfunction. *Am J Cardiol* 1997; **79**: 1670–73.

101. Christensen JH, Gustenhoff P, Korup E et al. Effect of fish oil on heart rate variability in survivors of myocardial infarction: a double blind randomised controlled trial. *BMJ* 1996; **312**: 677–8.

102. Christensen JH, Skou HA, Fog L et al. Marine n-3 fatty acids, wine intake, and heart rate variability in patients referred for coronary angiography. *Circulation* 2001; **103**: 651–7.

103. Christensen JH, Christensen MS, Dyerberg J, Schmidt EB. Heart rate variability and fatty acid content of blood cell membranes: a dose-response study with n-3 fatty acids. *Am J Clin Nutr* 1999; **70**: 331–7.

104. Christensen JH, Gustenhoff P, Ejlersen E et al. n-3 Fatty acids and ventricular extrasystoles in patients with ventricular tachyarrhythmias. *Nutr Res* 1995; **15**: 1–8.

105. Vreugdenhil M, Bruehl C, Voskuyl RA et al. Polyunsaturated fatty acids modulate sodium and calcium currents in CA1 neurons. *Proc Natl Acad Sci USA* 1996; **93**: 12 559–63.

106. Voskuyl RA, Vreugdenhil M, Kang JX, Leaf A. Anticonvulsant effect of polyunsaturated fatty acids in rats, using the cortical stimulation model. *Eur J Pharmacol* 1998; **341**: 145–52.

107. McLennan PL, Abeywardena MY, Charnock JS. Influence of dietary lipids on arrhythmias and infarction after coronary artery ligation in rats. *Can J Physiol Pharmacol* 1985; **63**: 1411–17.

108. McLennan PL, Abeywardena MY, Charnock JS. Dietary fish oil prevents ventricular fibrillation following coronary artery occlusion and reperfusion. *Am Heart J* 1988; **116**: 709–17.

109. McLennan PL. Relative effects of dietary saturated, monounsaturated, and polyunsaturated fatty acids on cardiac arrhythmias in rats. *Am J Clin Nutr* 1993; **57**: 207–12.

110. Charnock JS. Dietary fats and cardiac arrhythmia in primates. *Nutrition* 1994; **10**: 161–9.

111. McLennan PL, Bridle TM, Abeywardena MY, Charnock JS. Dietary lipid modulation of ventricular fibrillation threshold in the marmoset monkey. *Am Heart J* 1992; **123**: 1555–61.

112. Al Makdessi S, Brändle M, Ehrt M et al. Myocardial protection by ischemic preconditioning: the influence of the composition of myocardial phospholipids. *Mol Cell Biochem* 1995; **145**: 69–73.

113. Billman GE, Kang JX, Leaf A. Prevention of sudden cardiac death by dietary pure ω-3 polyunsaturated fatty acids in dogs. *Circulation* 1999; **99**: 2452–7.

114. Billman GE, Kang JX, Leaf A. Prevention of ischemia-induced cardiac sudden death by n-3 polyunsaturated fatty acids in dogs. *Lipids* 1997; **32**: 1161–8.

115. Billman GE, Hallaq H, Leaf A. Prevention of ischemia-induced ventricular fibrillation by ω3 fatty acids. *Proc Natl Acad Sci USA* 1994; **91**: 4427–30.

116. Nair SSD, Leitch JW, Falconer J, Garg ML. Prevention of cardiac arrhythmia by dietary (n-3) polyunsaturated fatty acids and their mechanism of action. *J Nutr* 1997; **127**: 383–93.

117. Kang JX, Leaf A. Antiarrhythmic effects of polyunsaturated fatty acids. Recent studies. *Circulation* 1996; **94**: 1774–80.

118. Weylandt KH, Kang JX, Leaf A. Polyunsaturated fatty acids exert antiarrhythmic actions as free acids rather than in phospholipids. *Lipids* 1996; **31**: 977–82.

119. Leaf A. The electrophysiological basis for the antiarrhythmic actions of polyunsaturated fatty acids. *Eur Heart J Suppl* 2001; **3(suppl D)**: D98–105.

120. Pound EM, Kang JX, Leaf A. Partitioning of polyunsaturated fatty acids, which prevent cardiac arrhythmias, into phospholipid cell membranes. *J Lipid Res* 2001; **42**: 346–51.

121. Rosenberg IH. Fish – food to calm the heart. *N Engl J Med* 2002; **346**: 1102–3.

122. Leaf A, Kang JX. Prevention of cardiac sudden death by N-3 fatty acids: a review of the evidence. *J Intern Med* 1996; **240**: 5–12.

123. Kang JX, Leaf A. Prevention of fatal cardiac arrhythmias by polyunsaturated fatty acids. *J Am Clin Nutr* 2000; **71**: 202–7.

124. Kang JX, Leaf A. Evidence that free polyunsaturated fatty acids modify Na+ channels by directly binding to the channel proteins. *Proc Natl Acad Sci USA* 1996; **93**: 3542–6.

125. Kang JX, Li Y, Leaf A. Regulation of sodium channel gene expression by class I antiarrhythmic drugs and n-3 polyunsaturated fatty acids in cultured neonatal rat cardiac myocytes. *Proc Natl Acad Sci USA* 1997; **94**: 2724–8.

126. Catterall WA. Structure and function of voltage-sensitive ion channels. *Science* 1988; **242**: 50–61.

127. Hallaq H, Smith TW, Leaf A. Modulation of dihydropyridine-sensitive calcium channels in heart cells by fish oil fatty acids. *Proc Natl Acad Sci USA* 1992; **89**: 1760–64.

128. Hallaq H, Sellmayer A, Smith TW, Leaf A. Protective effect of eicosapentaenoic acid on ouabain toxicity in neonatal rat cardiac myocytes. *Proc Natl Acad Sci USA* 1990; **87**: 7834–8.

129. Xiao Y-F, Gomez AM, Morgan JP et al. Suppression of voltage-gated L-type Ca^{2+} currents by polyunsaturated fatty acids in adult and neonatal rat ventricular myocytes. *Proc Natl Acad Sci USA* 1997; **94**: 4182–7.

130. Pepe S, Bogdanov K, Hallaq H et al. ω3 Polyunsaturated fatty acid modulates dihydropyridine effects on L-type Ca^{2+} channels, cytosolic Ca^{2+} and contraction in adult rat cardiac myocytes. *Proc Natl Acad Sci USA* 1994; **91**: 8832–6.

131. Pepe S, McLennan PL. Cardiac membrane fatty acid composition modulates myocardial oxygen consumption and postischemic recovery of contractile function. *Circulation* 2002; **105**: 2303–8.

132. Honoré E, Barhanin J, Attali B et al. External blockade of the major cardiac delayed-rectifier K+ channel (Kv1.5) by polyunsaturated fatty acids. *Proc Natl Acad Sci USA* 1994; **91**: 1937–44.

133. Singh RB, Niaz MA, Kartik C. Can n-3 fatty acids provide myocardial protection by decreasing infarct size and inhibiting atherothrombosis? *Eur Heart J Suppl* 2001; **3(suppl D)**: D62–9.

134. Meydani SN, Endres S, Woods MM et al. Oral (n-3) fatty acid supplementation suppresses cytokine production

and lymphocyte proliferation: comparison between young and older women. *J Nutr* 1991; **121**: 547–55.

135. Meydani SN, Lichtenstein AH, Cornwall S *et al*. Immunologic effects of National Cholesterol Education Panel step-2 diets with and without fish-derived N-3 fatty acid enrichment. *J Clin Invest* 1993; **92**: 105–13.

136. Von Schacky C. n-3 Fatty acids and the prevention of coronary atherosclerosis. *Am J Clin Nutr* 2000; **71(suppl)**: 224S–7S.

137. Von Schacky C. Dietary omega-3 fatty acids and human growth factor and cytokine gene expression. *Eur Heart J Suppl* 2001; **3(suppl D)**: D50–52.

138. Chin JPF. Marine oils and cardiovascular reactivity. *Prostaglandins Leukot Essent Fatty Acids* 1994; **50**: 211–22.

139. Mehta J, Lawson D, Saldeen T. Reduction in plasminogen activator inhibitor-1 (PAI-1) with omega-3 polyunsaturated fatty acid (PUFA) intake. *Am Heart J* 1988; **116**: 1201–6.

140. Saynor R, Verel D, Gillott T. The long-term effect of dietary supplementation with fish lipid concentrate on serum lipids, bleeding time, platelets and angina. *Atherosclerosis* 1984; **50**: 3–10.

141. Brown AJ, Roberts DCK. Fish and fish oil intake: effect on haematological variables related to cardiovascular disease. *Thromb Res* 1991; **64**: 169–78.

142. Von Schacky C, Angerer P, Kothny W *et al*. The effect of dietary ω-3 fatty acids on coronary atherosclerosis. A randomized, double-blind, placebo-controlled trial. *Ann Intern Med* 1999; **130**: 554–62.

143. Bairati I, Roy L, Meyer F. Double-blind, randomized, controlled trial of fish oil supplements in prevention of recurrence of stenosis after coronary angioplasty. *Circulation* 1992; **85**: 950–56.

144. Johansen O, Brekke M, Seljeflot I *et al*. n-3 Fatty acids do not prevent restenosis after coronary angioplasty: results from the CART study. *J Am Coll Cardiol* 1999; **33**: 1619–26.

145. Diep QN, Touyz RM, Schiffrin EL. Docosahexaenoic acid, a peroxisome proliferator-activated receptor-α ligand, induces apoptosis in vascular smooth muscle cells by stimulation of p38 mitogen-activated protein kinase. *Hypertension* 2000; **36**: 851–5.

146. Harris WS, Ginsberg HN, Arunakul N *et al*. Safety and efficacy of Omacor in severe hypertriglyceridemia. *J Cardiovasc Risk* 1997; **4**: 385–91.

147. Bhatnagar D, Mackness MI, Durrington PN. Treatment of mixed hyperlipidaemia using a combination of omega-3 fatty acids and HMG CoA reductase inhibitor. *Eur Heart J Suppl* 2001; **3(suppl D)**: D53–8.